**This book is to be returned on or before
the last date stamped below.**

Diagnosis before First Aid

Diagnosis before First Aid
A Manual for Emergency Care Workers

Neville Marsden
M.R.C.S., L.R.C.P., D.Obst. R.C.O.G.
General Practitioner; Clinical Assistant, accident and emergency
department, Victoria Hospital, Burnley;
Chairman of Rossendale Fell Rescue Team.

Foreword by
Noel F. Kirkman, M.D., F.R.C.S.
Honorary Consultant Surgeon at the University of South Manchester;
Chairman of the Mountain Rescue Committee of England and Wales.

CHURCHILL LIVINGSTONE
EDINBURGH LONDON AND NEW YORK 1978

CHURCHILL LIVINGSTONE
Medical Division of Longman Group Limited

Distributed in the United States of America by
Churchill Livingstone Inc., 19 West 44th Street,
New York, N.Y. 10036 and by associated
companies, branches and representatives
throughout the world.

First published 1978
  Reprinted 1980

ISBN 0 443 01639 9

British Library Cataloguing in Publication Data

Marsden, Neville
  Diagnosis before first aid.
  1. First aid in illness and injury   2. Diagnosis
  I. Title
  614.8'8   RC87

Printed in Singapore by
Singapore Offset Printing (Pte) Ltd.

Foreword

Despite the variety of first aid manuals available, this book fills a vacant niche because of its fresh and occasionally unorthodox style and the insistence of as good a diagnosis as possible in the field. This emphasis on diagnosis as a prerequisite for satisfactory first aid is highly commendable.

Dr Neville Marsden's exposition of the head to toe examination of casualties in a systematic way and his recurrent reiteration of the importance of comparing the injured to the uninjured part or side will be fully supported by all who teach first aid or work in a casualty department. The clear illustrations effectively emphasise many of the points made in the text. The first aider may perhaps save a life on some rare occasion if he has read and remembered the account of tracheotomy. Dr Marsden justly stresses the need to make every available effort to dislodge the foreign body obstructing the larynx before this heroic procedure is attempted.

This book is the outcome of many first aid courses which Dr Marsden has given to mountain rescue team members and other emergency care workers; it has been prompted by their problems and questions.

Although primarily written for the active first aider, this book could be read with profit by physiotherapists and medical students in the early years of their courses. It is a welcome addition to the literature on the constantly growing problems of first aid.

1977   Noel F. Kirkman, M.D., F.R.C.S.

Preface

Over a period of a few years, I have met First Aiders belonging to various organisations. I suppose that this was more or less inevitable since I have been a full-time casualty officer. I am now a part-time casualty officer, my main occupation being General Practice.

The first thing about First Aiders which impresses me, is their obvious enthusiasm for First Aid. The second thing which impresses me, is their desire to increase their own knowledge and ability.

It was their thirst for knowledge which prompted me to write this book. I would not have known what to write, without first finding out what the First Aiders wanted and needed to know, and I found this out through personal contact with them. I hope that I have provided the answers to their questions.

Lancashire, 1977   N.M.

Acknowledgements

For their reading and constructive criticism of the manuscript, I wish to express my thanks to Peter Durst, Leader of the Rossendale Fell Rescue Team, to Corporal Trevor Loftus, Deputy Leader of the R.A.F. (Stafford) Mountain Rescue Team, and last, but by no means least, to Dr A. S. G. ('Tony') Jones, Leader of the Ogwen Valley Mountain Rescue Team, in North Wales. By their comments and suggestions, all three have made valuable contributions to this book. I am further indebted to Trevor Loftus for all the diagrams and cartoons, and also to Henry Stott, Brian Veevers and Bryan Wilson (members of the Rossendale Fell Rescue Team), who helped a great deal towards the production of the diagrams of limb movements. I wish to thank Mrs Susan M. Dunning for typing the manuscript, and also the publishers, Churchill Livingstone, for their co-operation. Finally, for his foreword, I thank Mr Noel F. Kirkman; I am proud to count myself amongst his former students.

Contents

Introduction

This book is based on a series of talks given to the Rossendale Fell Rescue Team. The text is written in such a way as to give the impression that the author is speaking in person to the reader. This should make for easy reading of the text.

The objects of this book are to improve the First Aider's ability to diagnose and to improve the First Aider's understanding of the injured person. If a First Aider can achieve these two objectives, then he, or she, will be far more competent than before, when dealing with the single casualty, and will also be better able to decide correctly on the order of priority for evacuation, when dealing with mass casualties. Therefore, in order to concentrate attention on diagnosis, a great deal about treatment has been omitted purposely. Treatment is quite adequately dealt with in numerous books on First Aid. However, treatment varies from time to time, whereas diagnosis does not. A fractured clavicle is a fractured clavicle, whether it is treated by broad-arm sling, or by a figure-of-eight bandage.

First Aiders tend to concentrate on practising First Aid treatment such as splinting, bandaging and mouth-to-mouth respiration. This is *not* the logical approach to First Aid. *Diagnosis must always precede treatment.* Some injuries are obvious, but others are not. This book will teach the First Aider to search for those injuries which are not obvious. As he, or she, reads this book and *practises* what he, or she, is told to practise, it will become evident to the First Aider that the logical approach to any injured person is history, examination, diagnosis and *then* treatment.

The book is divided into Parts I, II and III. Please read them in that order. Part I is necessarily factual, and facts tend to be boring. However it is essential to read Part I thoroughly, if Parts II and III are to be understood properly. I have tried to include only the essential facts, without producing a whole textbook on human biology. Part II deals with History and Examination and in particular with the system of head-to-toe examination, which the First Aider is encouraged to practise as much as possible. It is an efficient method of examination. It saves time, eliminates doubt, and therefore, increases the First Aider's confidence. Part III deals with specific subjects.

I trust that the First Aider will enjoy this book, and that after reading it and practising what is preached, his, or her, diagnostic ability and understanding of the injured person will have improved considerably.

Part I: How Do We Function?

Diagnosis depends on our ability to recognise the abnormal. If we are to recognise the abnormal, then it is logical that we should first learn to know what is normal. Therefore, it is necessary to have a basic understanding of the normal functions of the human body before we proceed any further. In fact, it is so necessary, that medical students spend two years learning about the normal human body before they even begin to learn about illness and injury.

Basically, the human body is a living mechanism which needs energy for its function and survival. Energy is obtained by the combination of food products with oxygen in the tissues. The food products are obtained from the food we eat, and oxygen is obtained via the lungs. Both oxygen and the food products are transported to the tissues by the bloodstream, which also carries away the waste products of energy production from the tissues. These waste products are excreted via the lungs and kidneys. The food residue, which is the unuseable part of the food we eat, is eliminated as faeces.

The cell

This is the basic unit of the body. We are composed of millions upon millions of cells, which are so small that they can be seen only with the aid of a microscope. There are many different types of cell. It is not necessary for the First Aider to know them all. It is sufficient to say that each cell of the body has its own particular function to perform and it is constructed appropriately. For example, the red and white cells of the blood are rounded to facilitate travel within the bloodstream, whereas the cells which form the inner linings of the blood vessels are very thin, flat and smooth to prevent turbulent blood-flow, which could lead to the formation of a blood clot. Muscle cells can vary their length; they can contract or relax. On the other hand, nerve cells cannot vary their length. They transmit nerve impulses from one part of the body to another. A nerve cell may be very long indeed but if it is stretched it will be damaged. So, every cell has its own special function to perform and it contributes to the function of the human body as a whole.

The alimentary system

The word 'alimentary' simply means the mouth, throat, gullet, stomach, small intestine, large intestine, rectum and anus, in that order. It is the food-tube which passes right through us from one end to the other. Food is chewed in the mouth and swallowed down the gullet into the stomach, where it is churned up by the muscular action of the stomach and partly broken down by the stomach's acid juice. From the stomach the food is passed into the small intestine, where a number of chemical juices break it down into its basic components, *viz*:

1. Carbohydrates – i.e. sugars, e.g. from bread and potatoes.
2. Fatty acids – these are the basic components of fats.
3. Amino acids – Sorry, but there is no other name for these. Amino acids are the basic chemical 'bricks' used to build up proteins.

When the food has been broken down into these food products, it is passed along the bowel by rhythmic bowel movements, and these movements give rise to *bowel sounds,* which can be heard by placing your ear to someone else's abdomen. *Try it.* You will need to listen for bowel sounds later, when you come to examine the abdomen, so you may as well get used to recognising normal bowel sounds *now*!

Eventually, the food products are absorbed through the bowel wall, and they are taken, via the bloodstream and the lymphatic vessels, to the liver for storage. From the liver, the sugars can be sent (as glucose) to the muscles, via the bloodstream, to be used for energy production. The amino acids can be sent to any part of the body to be built up into new proteins, which will replace old, worn-out proteins. The fats are stored all over the body in fat depots. A very important fat depot is the fat deposited under the skin. This helps to insulate the body against the cold. Fats are also a reserve supply of energy, although energy can be obtained much more rapidly from glucose.

The unwanted by-products of digestion are known as the food residue. This is passed into the large bowel, where as much water as possible is absorbed from it. This is one of the body's *fluid-conservation mechanisms.* (These mechanisms are important and will be referred to again). The remainder of the food residue is passed out through the anus at intervals as faeces (i.e. 'stools').

The above is a very brief description of the function of the human digestive system. Just how brief it is can be judged by the fact that research workers can spend a whole lifetime studying it. Let us now consider the body's use of the sugars, etc., which it has acquired from plants or from other animals.

Metabolism

Metabolism is simply a word which, in a nutshell, means, 'The production and use of energy'. Thus, we can use one word instead of six; it saves time, and besides that, later on, I shall refer to something called the metabolic rate. (The metabolic rate is the *rate* of production and use of energy). We use energy for all our activities, and one very important activity is to maintain our body temperatures at the correct level of 37°C

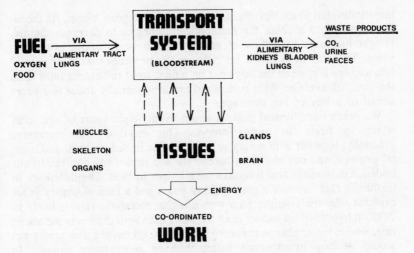

Fig. 1

(98.6°F), or slightly below this. If our body temperature falls to 25°C (77°F), we are well and truly in a state of hypothermia, and if it falls to 20°C (68°F) we will die. So, in order to stay alive and healthy, we must maintain a body temperature of 37°C (98.6°F). Our muscles use energy when we move about, or even when we stand still, because in standing still, our muscle-actions are balancing each other, so that we do not fall over. The heart uses energy to pump blood around the circulatory system. In fact, every cell which goes to make up the human body uses energy, and in order to produce energy the following processes may occur:

1. Glucose reacts with oxygen to produce water, carbon dioxide and energy.

2. Fats can be broken down slowly to produce water, carbon dioxide and energy.

3. Proteins can be broken down to give urea, water, carbon dioxide and energy.

The exact methods by which these processes occur are very complicated indeed, but it is not necessary for you to know exactly how they work. It is quite sufficient for you to know that these three mechanisms of energy-production exist.

The metabolic rate varies according to age, build and sex. Babies have a high metabolic rate, because they have to grow from about 7 lbs (3.55 kg) at birth to about 28 lbs (14.2 kg) at the age of twelve months. Babies are particularly vulnerable to hypothermia, because they can burn up their energy reserves very rapidly. Therefore, babies have to be well clothed, to prevent excessive heat loss, and they have to be fed more times per day than adults in order to keep up their energy supplies. A young baby's main occupation is sleeping, because the baby's energy is largely devoted to multiplying its cells, in order to grow bigger. As the infant grows into a child, the metabolic rate begins to decrease slightly. Height increases by spurts of growth, which occur about every two years. The growth in height by girls usually precedes that of boys until late teenage life, when the boys put on a final spurt to become taller than the girls, on average. As a rule, a girl matures sexually about two years ahead of a boy of her own age.

We reach our physical peak at about twenty-eight years of age, after which we begin the *ageing process*. Our metabolic rate decreases gradually, together with a very gradual decline in our physical and mental prowess and our ability to regenerate and repair any damage to our bodies, i.e. wounds and fractures take longer to heal. The difference in metabolic rate between a man of forty years and a man of twenty years explains why the younger man with a higher metabolic rate, is likely to develop hypothermia sooner than the older man with the lower metabolic rate, who is better able to conserve his energy. Likewise a slim young girl would develop hypothermia faster than an older fatter woman. In general, women can resist hypothermia better than men do because:

    a. they tend to have a lower metabolic rate, and

    b. they have a thicker layer of fat underneath the skin, which gives them better insulation against the cold, than men have.

Excretion and kidney function

Excretion is the process by which the unwanted by-products of metabolism are eliminated from the body, i.e. excess water, excess carbon dioxide and urea. *Carbon dioxide,* produced by cell metabolism, passes into the blood, which transports it to the lungs from where it is passed out of the body with the expired air. However, carbon dioxide, when dissolved in water forms a bicarbonate ion, which can be excreted by the kidneys *selectively.* The kidneys can regulate the amount of bicarbonate ions excreted, and this is important in maintaining the correct pH of the body. (This will be explained later.) *Urea* is a completely harmless by-product of protein metabolism and it is of no further use to the body. Therefore, the kidneys simply excrete it as it reaches them, via the bloodstream. *Water* is a very necessary substance for our existence. In fact, about 60 per cent of our total body weight is water. It is possible for a human being to survive for about one month on fresh water alone and no food; but without water we can survive only a few days. Even so, it is necessary to have the right amount of water in us, and any excess is excreted by the kidneys. Water can also be lost by sweating, and as water vapour (small amounts) in the expired air.

The kidneys perform their functions by acting as elaborate filtering mechanisms. About one fifth of the blood pumped out by the heart in any given minute passes through the kidneys. As the blood passes through the kidneys, a fair volume of the plasma is filtered into tiny tubes. These tiny tubes (or tubules) reabsorb water, glucose and the mineral elements required by the body, whilst at the same time not reabsorbing urea. The tubules are highly selective in their ability to reabsorb (or not to reabsorb) the chemical substances which filter through to them, and are therefore able to regulate the chemical balance of the body fluids. For the chemically minded First Aiders, the body fluids must be kept slightly alkaline; i.e. they must be kept within a range of pH of 7.2 – 7.6 (average pH 7.4). Any variation outside this range is *lethal* to human beings.

For the non-chemically minded First Aiders, I should explain that pH is a term used to describe acidity or alkalinity, e.g. pH 1.0 means that a substance is very strongly acid; pH 12.0 means that a substance is very strongly alkaline and pH 7.0 is neutral.

The kidney functions, therefore, are extremely delicate and complicated, but they can be summarised briefly as follows:

1. Excretion of urea (and other substances no longer required).
2. Reabsorption of glucose (and other substances required).
3. Regulation of pH.
4. Regulation of chemical composition of body fluids.
5. Reabsorption of water, i.e. *fluid conservation* (except for the amount of water necessary to form urine).

Once the urine is formed, it passes from the kidneys, down the ureters to the bladder, where it is stored. At intervals, the bladder is emptied by passing the urine to the outside world, via the urethra.

Circulation, respiration and blood pressure

The heart is the strong muscular pump which pushes the blood round the whole circulatory system. Blood is pumped through the lungs, where carbon dioxide passes out of the blood into the air sacs of the lungs. At the same time, oxygen passes from the air sacs of the lungs into the blood. In fact, it is the haemoglobin inside the red cells of the blood, which carries carbon dioxide to the lungs and oxygen away from the lungs. The oxygen is acquired by inhaling and the carbon dioxide is expelled by exhaling. When the blood reaches the tissues the reverse happens – the red cells give up their oxygen, which passes into the tissue cells, and the tissue cells give up carbon dioxide, which passes into the red cells. This whole process is called *respiration*.

After passing through the lungs, the blood returns to the heart and it is then distributed to the rest of the body via the aorta. The aorta gives off smaller arteries, which in turn give off even smaller arteries, until a system of tiny vessels called *arterioles* is reached. The arteries have *elastic* walls, and are therefore capable of expansion and recoil (it is the expansion of the radial artery, for example, which you can feel in the pulse at the wrist). The arterioles, however, are important little blood vessels, because they have *muscular* walls. This enables them to control the flow of blood through them, because each arteriole can alter its calibre. If an arteriole constricts, it will reduce the amount of blood passing through it, but if it dilates (by relaxing its muscular wall), it will increase the amount of blood flowing through it. *Therefore, the amount of blood-flow to any part of the body at any particular time is determined by the state of constriction, or dilation, of the arterioles in that part of the body at that particular time.* This is a very important fact. When we are at rest after a meal, the arterioles controlling blood supply to the gut open up, because our digestive processes are at work, but the arterioles to our muscles tend to shut down, because we are resting. When we are running, working etc., the reverse occurs. In other words, our arterioles enable us to send blood to the places which most need it at any given time.

After passing through the arterioles, the blood enters a system of microscopic vessels in the tissues called *capillaries*, and it is here that the cells exchange carbon dioxide for a fresh supply of oxygen. The blood then enters a system of minute *venules*, which merge to form *veins*, which in turn, merge to form larger veins until the blood finally reaches the heart via the vena cava, and the whole process is repeated.

Blood pressure

As the heart pushes blood around the circulatory system, the blood is under a certain amount of pressure. If the blood was not under any pressure at all, then it would not move, would it? When the heart contracts (i.e. pumps), we call the period of contraction *systole*, and the period during which the heart relaxes is called *diastole*. So, when the heart pumps blood out into the Aorta, the blood pressure rises to a peak which is known as the *systolic blood pressure*. When the heart relaxes, the blood pressure falls to a basic level, called the *diastolic blood pressure*.

A typical systolic blood pressure would be 120 mmHg, and a typical diastolic blood pressure would be 70 mmHg. This would be recorded as, 'B.P. _ $\frac{120}{70}$ '. The blood pressure varies from one individual to another, but the accepted normal maximum readings are 140 mmHg for the systolic and 90 mmHg for the diastolic blood pressure. The instrument used to measure blood pressure is called a sphygmomanometer (or 'sphyg.' for brevity). A description of the sphygmomanometer and how to use it will be given in Section II.

Before we leave this topic, I will clarify what is meant by the term *Pulse Pressure*. This is simply the difference between the systolic and diastolic blood pressures. So, take away the diastolic from the systolic blood pressure and you have the pulse pressure, e.g.:

1. B.P. = $\frac{120}{70}$ Therefore, pulse pressure = 120–70 = 50 mmHg
2. B.P. = $\frac{140}{80}$ Therefore, pulse pressure = 140–80 = 60 mmHg

Incidentally, the blood pressure is *always* measured in terms of millimeters of mercury (mmHg).

The adrenal glands

These are two small, pyramid-shaped glands which lie above the kidneys (one adrenal gland above each kidney). For this reason, they are sometimes called the suprarenal glands ('supra' = above; 'renal' = appertaining to the kidney). Each gland consists of a central part called the medulla, which produces a chemical substance called epinephrine. This is a mixture of adrenaline and noradrenaline. The outer part of the gland is called the cortex, and this produces Cortisone and other related chemicals.

During exercise, epinephrine is released into the circulation. It causes an increase in heart rate and pulse pressure and in the rate at which the blood circulates, because extra supplies of glucose and oxygen are needed by the muscles. If we are startled, or injured, adrenaline is suddenly injected into the circulation by the adrenal glands, and this causes a sudden increase in heart rate. This explains why you can feel your heart pounding when you are startled or frightened. In fact, a good way to remember the effects of the *adrenaline response* as it is called, is to say that it prepares us for *Fright, Fight and Flight.* Another effect of the adrenaline response is to reduce our ability to feel pain. This is just as important as it is logical. For instance, if an animal is injured in a fight, is losing the fight, and decides that there is no future in continuing the fight, then it breaks off the engagement and runs away. This is 'Flight', and obviously, during its flight for safety, it does not wish its ability to run to be impaired by pain. Adrenaline provides this lowered pain sensibility. The animal feels the pain later, when it has reached safety, and when the adrenaline response has worn off. Exactly the same response occurs in human beings, and it is important to remember this, because a fracture may remain painless for a few hours after injury, as a result of the adrenaline response. I remember well a man who had broken both wrists in a car crash. His face was pale because of the adrenaline response (i.e. 'Fright') and he could not use his hands because of the fractures, but he felt no pain. Even by moving the fractures so that I caused 'bony crepitus', (see *Injuries to Bones and Joints*) I could not cause him to feel pain. It was only six hours after the injury, when the adrenaline response wore off, that he began to feel any pain at all!

The blood

Basically, blood is a fluid composed of water, minerals, glucose, proteins, red blood cells and white blood cells. If we remove the red and white cells from the blood, the remaining fluid is plasma. Plasma is a very useful substance, because it can be dried and converted into a solid, just as milk can be converted to a powder. When a patient reaches hospital and needs an urgent transfusion of blood, a sample of his blood must be sent to the laboratory for cross-matching with the blood which is to be given to him. This is to ensure that his blood will not clot the red cells of the blood transfused into him. If that happened, the results would be disastrous. The cross-matching of blood can take up to one and a half hours, and this could be too long a delay for the patient. This is where the dried plasma can play a great role. By mixing the dried plasma with sterile water, the plasma becomes fluid again. It does not have to be cross-matched, can be given to the patient straight away and results in a marked improvement in the patient's general condition. Dried plasma can be stored for years and is reconstituted in two minutes.

The functions of the various constituents of the blood are as follows:

1. *Red cells*. These carry oxygen from the lungs to the tissues, and carbon dioxide from the tissues to the lungs.

2. *White cells*. These fight invading bacteria, and have certain other functions.

3. *Proteins*. These have three basic functions:

a. Clotting. A whole series of proteins take part in the clotting mechanism, which is very complex indeed.

b. Antibodies. These are the proteins which neutralise the poisons produced by bacteria.

c. Viscosity of the blood, i.e. the proteins help to keep the blood at its correct 'stickiness'. They stop it from becoming too watery.

4. *Chemical substances*. The main chemical substances in the blood are Sodium ions, Potassium ions, Chloride ions and Bicarbonate ions. The relative concentrations of these ions are delicately balanced in order to maintain the correct pH of the body (see *Kidney Function*, p. 4).

5. *Water*. This is the constituent which keeps the blood fluid.

The skin

The skin is divided basically into two main layers, the epidermis and the dermis.

1. *The epidermis*. This is the outside, or superficial layer. It has about five layers of cells. The deepest layer of cells is called the germinal layer. It produces cells which are pushed towards the surface. As the cells approach the surface they die, become flattened and eventually they flake off. This flattened, dead layer of cells forms a barrier, which is impervious to water. In other words, we have found yet another *fluid-conservation mechanism*. In fact, but for this water-impervious layer in our skins, we would all walk around dripping fluid at such a rate that we would not be able to drink water fast enough to replace the fluid lost!

2. *The dermis*. This is the deeper layer of the skin. Unlike the epidermis, it has a good supply of blood vessels. It also has hair follicles, from which hairs grow out beyond the skin surface. The sweat glands also originate in the dermis, as do the sebaceous glands, which secrete an oily substance onto the surface of the skin. Beneath the dermis there is a layer of fat.

Let us summarise the functions of the skin:

a. It offers a certain amount of protection to underlying structures.
b. It conserves fluid.
c. It produces sebaceous fluid which:
    i. helps to stop the skin from drying up;
    ii. discourages unwanted bacteria from inhabiting the skin because it is alkaline;
    iii. lubricates the bases of the hairs, so that they bend rather than break.
d. *Temperature regulation.* This is a very important function. When the body is becoming over-heated, the blood vessels in the dermis dilate. This increases the blood-flow near the surface of the body. Since blood is warm, this means that there is more heat available for direct radiation to the surface of the body and then away to the atmosphere. If this does not get rid of enough excess heat, then the sweat glands come into operation. They secrete a film of very dilute salt solution (sweat) onto the surface of the skin. When the film of sweat evaporates from the body surface, then (in accordance with the laws of physics) heat is lost from the body surface.

When the temperature of our surroundings falls below a certain level, the blood vessels in the dermis reduce heat loss to a minimum by constricting themselves and reducing the blood-flow through the dermis to a minute quantity. However, this constriction of blood vessels in the dermis cannot last indefinitely, otherwise the skin itself would die from lack of nourishment. So, eventually the vessels in the dermis must re-dilate, and when they do so, they over-dilate in order to compensate for the time during which the skin has been relatively undernourished. This compensatory over-dilation is called *reactive hyperaemia* – just think of how pink your fingers become when you warm your hands in front of the fire, after being out on a cold winter's day! Now, this reactive hyperaemia is perfectly natural and safe, *provided* that we have found a place of shelter and warmth. However, if someone becomes extremely deeply hypothermic, without finding shelter, and if his skin vessels cannot constrict any longer, then reactive hyperaemia will occur, giving him the sensation of a warm glow all over, but he will die quickly, owing to the rapid heat-loss which will ensue.

Body fluids

I have made mention of fluid-conservation mechanisms already. Let us now list the organs involved in fluid-conservation. They are:

1. The skin (impervious to water).
2. The kidneys (they lose only as much water as is necessary to form urine).
3. The large bowel (it absorbs as much fluid as possible from the food residue).

If the kidneys or the large bowel are malfunctioning then there is nothing much that the First Aider can do about it. However, I would like to stress at this point, that *a great deal of fluid can be lost from a superficial burn*, i.e. from a burn which has destroyed only the superficial, water-impervious layer of the skin, leaving the dermis intact. I have actually seen half a pint of plasma drip from a superficial burn on a man's forearm in a matter of only ten minutes. At that rate, he would have lost three pints of fluid in one hour! The treatment for this kind of burn is to cover up the burn (as instructed in the First Aid Manuals) and to cover the dressing with a good, *firm* bandage. The principle involved here is that the pressure of the bandage should exceed the pressure under which the plasma is oozing through the surface of the burn, and this should reduce fluid loss to a minimum.

Let us now turn our attention to the distribution of the body fluids. As stated before, about 60 per cent of the human body is composed of fluid. Most of this fluid is inside the cells and is known as Intracellular Fluid (ICF). All the fluid which is outside the cells is known as Extracellular Fluid (ECF). From a strictly technical viewpoint, ECF includes blood, since blood is outside the tissue cells. From a purely practical point of view, it is better to regard blood as a separate fluid from the rest of the ECF. So, in this book, whenever the term 'ECF' is used, it will refer to all of the extracellular fluid, excluding the blood. The reason for this will soon become apparent.

In general, women have slightly less fluid per kilogram of body weight than men. The body fluids of a man who weighs 70 kg (11 stones) can be summarised as follows:

	Litres		Pints (approx.)
Total blood volume	=	4.92	8½
ECF (excluding blood)	=	6.08	10½
ICF	=	32.00	56½
Total body fluids	=	43.00	75½

The practical importance of ECF

It is the human equivalent of the hump on the camel's back. In other words, it is a valuable reserve of fluid for emergencies. This applies particularly when blood is lost. Reserves of fluid can be drawn from the ECF, via the capillaries, into the blood vessels in order to make up for the volume of blood lost, although ECF can never make up for the loss of red cells. This ability to replenish blood volume after blood loss, prevents the heart from going into failure (which would happen if the blood volume continued to decline). So, it can be appreciated that if this store of ECF did not exist, then many people would not live long enough after injury to reach hospital and be transfused. In fact, many people, now alive after injury, would be dead. These people owe their lives to *blood transfu-*

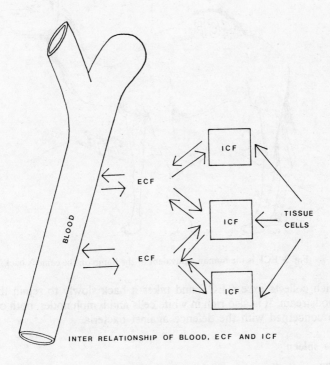

INTER RELATIONSHIP OF BLOOD, ECF AND ICF

Fig. 2

sion, because the only real replacement for blood is blood.

The existence of ECF, and its function during emergencies, creates a valuable time interval for casualties after injury. Please remember that *THIS TIME IS VALUABLE*, and it should never be wasted. There is a limit to the amount of ECF which can be drawn into the bloodstream, and there is a limit to the number of red cells which the casualty can afford to lose. So, if an injured person needs blood, secure the airway, stop haemorrhage, spend no more time than is absolutely necessary on splinting and get him as quickly as possible to the place where blood is available – HOSPITAL!

The lymphatic system

This was mentioned briefly before in connection with the absorption of fats from the intestine. In fact, it is basically a separate vascular system,

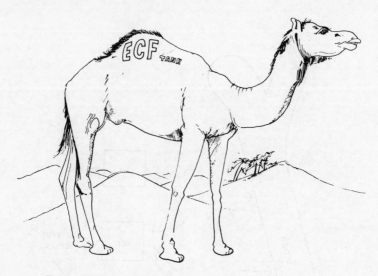

Fig. 3 'ECF is the human equivalent of the hump on the camel's back.'

which collects excess ECF and takes it back slowly to rejoin the main bloodstream. It is also rich in white cells and lymph nodes, both of which are concerned with the defence against bacteria.

The spleen

The entire functions of this organ are still not known. We do know that it contains a reserve supply of red cells, which it can inject into the circulation in an emergency, e.g. sudden heavy blood loss. Otherwise, as far as the First Aider is concerned, the spleen exists in order to be injured!

The nervous system

You do not need a detailed knowledge of this. *Sensory impulses*, e.g. touch, pain, pressure — from all parts of the body (skin, muscles, joints etc.) travel along the nerves towards the spinal cord and then up the spinal cord to the brain. *Motor impulses* originating in the brain (and usually triggered off by the arrival of a sensory impulse) travel down the spinal cord and out along the nerves to the muscles, which, being stimulated by the motor impulse, then contract. This is a very simple explanation of the basic way in which the nervous system works.

Some impulses reach conscious level (e.g. pain), but there are many which do not. For example, when you are standing, you are aware that you are standing but you are not aware of the hundreds of nervous impulses shooting up and down the spinal cord in order to keep you standing. The same applies to walking. When you wish to walk, you walk;

but what you are not aware of is the fact that every step involves hundreds of nervous impulses, and muscle and joint movements. If we had to initiate from *conscious* level every nervous impulse necessary to enable us to walk, then life would be very slow and difficult indeed!

There are two other important factors which I should mention. The first is, that the right side of the cerebrum (brain) controls the movements of the left side of the body, and vice versa. This is useful to remember when dealing with someone who has had a stroke. The second important factor is that the *speech centre* in right-handed people is in the left cerebrum. In left-handed people it is in the right cerebrum. Therefore, if a right-handed person has a stroke in the right cerebrum, causing paralysis in the left arm and leg, then he will still be able to speak, although his speech may be affected by weakness of the left side of the face. If a right-handed person has a stroke in the left cerebrum (affecting the right arm and leg), then he will almost certainly lose his ability to speak coherently, because the speech centre is almost invariably affected. For a left-handed person, the situations are reversed.

The bones

The bones of a living person are *alive*. They maintain our shape by giving support to the softer tissues. The basic component of bone is a protein called *ossein*, and this protein is formed into the structure of each individual bone by bone-forming cells called *osteoblasts*. Calcium salts are deposited in the ossein in order to add rigidity to the bone. Old and damaged bone is removed by cells called *osteoclasts*, which thus make way for the osteoblasts to move in and lay down new bone. This process of renewal of bone goes on constantly throughout our lives. If it did not occur, then spontaneous fractures would occur when bones had been in use for a certain length of time, just as fatigue fractures can occur in metals, which have been in service for a long time.

Since bone is a living substance, every bone has a blood supply of its own. Therefore, when a bone is broken, the blood vessels in it are torn and blood can then flow out of the bone fragments at the fracture site. This is an important fact. *Broken bones bleed*, and the amount of blood lost depends on which bone is broken. In general, the larger the bone, the greater the blood loss. Since the blood vessels in bones are relatively small, the blood is lost at a fairly slow rate, usually over a period of three hours or more; but the blood is lost from the circulation, just as surely as if it had poured out onto the ground. The estimate of blood loss from various bones is dealt with in Section III (*Injuries to Bones and Joints*).

Joints

There are different types of joint in the body, but those with which you are principally concerned are the joints of the limbs, and these are synovial joints. A synovial joint is formed between the ends of two or more bones. The bone ends are covered with a special kind of cartilage, called articular cartilage, which allows the bone ends to move smoothly against each other. The joint is surrounded by a tough capsule, inside which there is a delicate lining called the synovium. The synovium produces an oily fluid, called synovial fluid, which lubricates the joint.

The muscles

Muscles are composed of cells which can vary their length. When a muscle shortens (e.g. contracts) then the parts of the bones to which the muscle is attached, are brought closer to each other. In this way, the position of the joint between the two bones is altered. When the muscle relaxes, the joint is allowed to move the other way. Muscles are usually arranged in groups which work opposite each other, e.g. one group of muscles bends the elbow and the other group extends the elbow.

Having summarised the normal functions of the body, we can now start to learn how to diagnose the abnormal.

PART II: History and Examination

The history

When a doctor approaches a patient, the first thing he does is to ask questions. This is known, in the medical fraternity, as taking the history. The history can be divided into 'present' and 'previous' histories.

A. Present history

From a First Aider's point of view, the present history will almost always be concerned with an injury. Therefore, the following questions will be asked:

1. 'What happened?'
2. 'How did it happen?'
3. 'Where does it hurt?' (This gives a clue to the site or sites of injury.)
4. 'Have you been unconscious?' or 'Were you knocked out?'
5. 'Can you move your limbs and wiggle your toes?' (especially important when neck or back injury is suspected).

The above questions are a reasonable guide-line, but a word of caution to you. If somebody says, 'I fell,' then that is not enough. You must ask the following two questions: 'How far did you fall?' and 'How did you land?' There are two reasons for these two questions. Firstly, the farther a person falls, the worse his injuries are likely to be. Secondly, the part of the body which makes contact with the ground first is the part most likely to be injured. Having said that, I must state that it is common knowledge amongst orthopaedic surgeons (the 'bone and joint' surgeons) that if a man falls about twenty feet and lands on one or both feet, then, although the heels and ankles are the parts most likely to suffer, the force of the impact with the ground is transmitted upwards through the lower limbs to the pelvis and then continues up the spine to the base of the skull. It is therefore important to remember that, if a man falls twenty feet or more and lands on his feet, he may sustain fractures in any of the bones of the lower limbs, in the pelvis, the spinal bones or even in the base of the skull. This is a very important lesson to learn. So, remember the saying: 'The words, "I fell", should ring a bell.' This will remind you to ask how far the man fell and how he landed.

Question 4, 'Have you been unconscious?', is important, because in my experience, many people will not volunteer the fact that they have been unconscious. Perhaps they think that I know already, or perhaps they think that it does not matter now because they have recovered consciousness. Sometimes a person may not realise that he has been unconscious, in which case, the evidence of witnesses of the injury can be valuable. In any case, I always ask the question, just to make sure. Preferably, ask any witnesses *first* and then ask the patient. You will realise the importance of this when you read *Head Injuries*, in Part III.

B. Previous history

This can be of great importance. For example, if a person is unconscious and a friend is with him, it would be useful to know if the unconscious man is a known diabetic or epileptic. Similarly, if a man has had his right kidney removed at some time in the past, it would be foolish to make a diagnosis of rupture, or suspected rupture, of the right kidney in his case!

I have found that the least time-consuming approach to the previous history is to ask the following questions in this order:

1. 'Have you had any operations in the past?'
2. 'Have you ever had any serious illnesses?' (In relation to this question, I ask specifically if the person is diabetic or epileptic.)
3. 'Are you allergic to anything?' (In particular, I ask for allergy to penicillin, and for hay fever or asthma.)
4. In the case of a woman, I ask for previous obstetrical and gynaecological history − i.e. how many babies has she had, any miscarriages and any gynaecological operations. The First Aider will rarely find it necessary to go so deeply into a woman's previous history. However, it is possible that the First Aider may be faced with the task of delivering a baby, and when faced with the Emergency Childbirth Procedure, it is far more comforting to know that a woman has had three normal deliveries previously, than to know that she has had three previous Caesarean sections!

You may wonder why I ask the above questions in the above order. Well, there are many people who do not differentiate between illnesses and operations. After all, appendicitis is an illness, even though an operation may be necessary to cure it. However, an operation is a landmark in any person's medical history, because it takes place at a definite time. An illness may last for a variable time, from a few days up to a few months. Therefore by asking for operations first, we establish the landmarks, and at the same time, we isolate the previous surgical history (appendicectomy, etc.) from the previous medical history (pleurisy, duodenal ulcers, allergies, etc.) In any case, as I said before, I have found that this is the least time-consuming method of obtaining the previous history.

The information obtained from the history should be recorded as concisely as possible, because it can be of great value to the medical and nursing staff when the patient reaches hospital. In no case is this more true than in the case of a head injury history. Every scrap of information should be recorded, because the history may be the factor which determines whether or not the neurosurgeon has to operate.

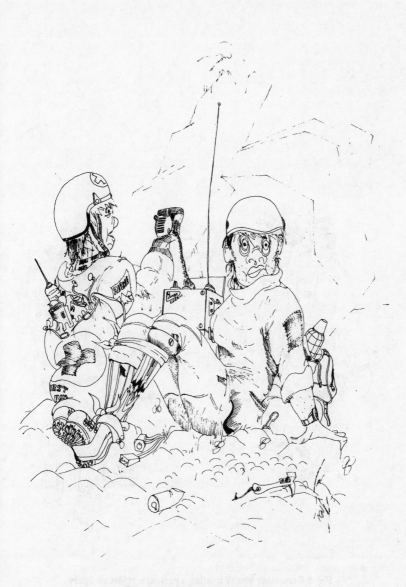

Fig. 4 Check the casualty's history.

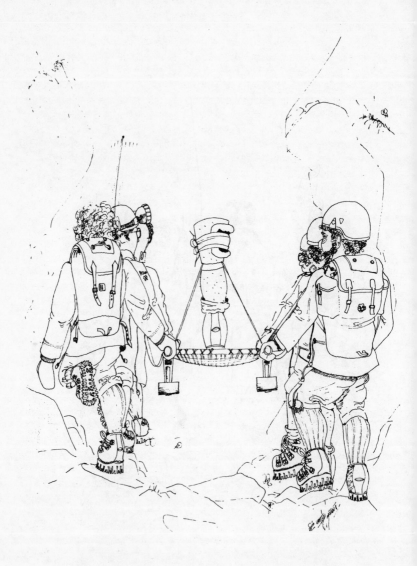

Fig. 5 Remember you're treating a person, not just an injury.

The examination

The basic method of examining a patient is a time-honoured sequence which, as any doctor can tell you, is inspection, palpation, percussion and auscultation, in that order. In other words, we use our eyes for looking (Inspection), our hands for feeling (Palpation), we drum on the patient's chest or abdomen and listen to the note produced (Percussion) and we listen to breath sounds and bowel sounds (Auscultation). It is a common myth that the doctor's stethoscope is a magical instrument. In fact, it is possible to hear breath sounds more clearly by putting the ear directly onto the chest (this is known as Direct Auscultation), than by using a stethoscope. Actually, the use of the stethoscope is rather more polite than direct auscultation (especially when the patient is a young lady!), and it saves the doctor from having to perform acrobatics in order to listen to a chest. Basically, therefore, when examining a patient, we are using the natural senses with which we have been endowed, i.e. sight, touch and hearing. Sometimes we even use our sense of smell. For instance, we can detect the sweet-smelling breath of a diabetic.

Once we have taken the history and examined the patient, we use the information so obtained, and we then arrive at a diagnosis. It is often stated that experience is a great teacher, and the more experience we gain, the more quickly we are able to arrive at a diagnosis. Let us proceed with the examination.

The general condition of the patient

It is one thing to diagnose individual injuries, but it must always be remembered that the injury is attached to a person, and not the other way around. In other words, you are treating a *person* all the time, no matter what the injury, or injuries, may be. The only reason for splinting a fractured limb is to make transportation more comfortable for the person to whom the limb belongs. With this in mind, we should always be aware of the general condition of the patient, because this will often be the determining factor in establishing priority of evacuation when dealing with mass casualties. It has been stated in many First Aid Manuals that the person who makes the most noise is the one who probably has the least injuries. This is often true, because he is still capable of devoting energy to a noisy display of anxiety. The person who is quiet, listless and often pale, is the one most likely to be seriously injured, because his energy is all being concentrated into trying to keep himself alive. He has no energy to spare for making a noise.

The five main factors which give us a good idea of the general condition of the patient are:
1. facial appearance
2. pulse
3. respiration

4. temperature
5. blood pressure.
I will deal with them in that order.

1. *Facial appearance*

An experienced person can often tell at a glance if a person is badly injured or not. For instance, if a person's facial colour is normal and he gives the appearance of being cool, calm, collected and alert, then the chances are that he is not badly injured, although it is well worth while making sure that he has not had a head injury. On the other hand, although someone who has sustained a head injury may have recovered consciousness and may appear quite alert, it is possible that he may have a far-away (or 'yonderly') look on his face. Someone who exhibits a pained expression is obviously in pain, while someone who has multiple injuries or who is very ill (e.g. pneumonia) may well a have 'cannot-be-bothered' expression, or an 'everything-is-too-much-trouble' expression. A flushed appearance may indicate an acute infection, or uncontrolled diabetes, and this may well be accompanied by deep rapid respiration (in diabetes), or rapid, shallow respiration, as in a pleurisy. Cyanosis (a bluish tinge of the lips) indicates that there is inadequate oxygenation of the blood and this may be due to a number of conditions, e.g. obstruction, or partial obstruction of the airway, heart disease or lung disease.

Someone who has lost three, or more, pints of blood would probably have a worried, anxious look on his face and would probably have a pale, cold and clammy skin. If the blood loss were greater than three pints, he would develop dark rings under his eyes, become restless and exhibit rapid, shallow breathing and would have a rapid, thready pulse. These signs indicate shock, and he would be in big trouble. If he were to go on to develop *Air Hunger* (i.e. deep, sighing respiration caused by gross loss of red blood cells), then he would be in very serious trouble, because he would surely die, if he were not transfused with blood very soon.

Shock is a clinical condition characterised by pallor, a cold, clammy skin and a rapid, thready pulse, and these three signs are associated with a lowering of blood pressure. The causes of shock can be divided into three groups *viz*:

1. Cardiogenic shock – i.e. anything which affects the function of the heart. Examples of this type of shock are coronary thrombosis, pneumothroax, stove-in-chest and electric shock.

2. Neurogenic shock – i.e. anything which affects nervous control over the heart and vascular system, especially pain. For example, the 'Acute Abdomen' (perforated duodenal ulcer, appendicitis, strangulated hernia, etc.) causes pain, which in turn causes shock.

3. Vascular shock. This is caused by heavy fluid loss, such as blood loss from fractures, internal bleeding, or external loss from a severed artery. Burns may result in heavy plasma loss, and sometimes cause gross destruction of red cells. Intestinal infections may cause profuse

vomiting or diarrhoea, resulting in a heavy loss of ECF, and heat stroke causes loss of ECF together with gross salt depletion. Vascular shock can be induced by any of these causes.

Pallor can also be the result of the adrenaline response to injury (this was mentioned in Part I). This form of pallor is usually associated with a *temporarily* raised blood pressure, and it occurs especially in young men within the first one to three hours after a serious injury. *Beware the pallor associated with a raised blood pressure after injury!* If the fracture is one from which three or more pints of blood can be lost, then eventually the blood pressure must come down to normal, and thereafter it will fall to below normal. Sometimes, the fall in blood pressure can be calamitously rapid, and therefore the injured person must have an intravenous drip set up as soon as possible (i.e. a sterile tube and needle put into a vein, to allow fluid to pass into his circulation). The reason for this is that, if his blood pressure does collapse suddenly, fluids can be pumped rapidly into his circulation to combat the fall in blood pressure.

Well, that more or less takes care of facial appearance, except for the comment that some bright spark somewhere must make, 'You cannot detect pallor in a dark-skinned person!' Well, hard luck, Mr Bright Spark, your statement is incorrect. A certain amount of pallor *can* be detected in the face of a coloured person, who is ill or injured, and this is true for the vast majority of coloured people. The exception to the rule is the coloured person whose skin looks *very* black indeed, but even then, pallor can be detected. Look at the fingernails. Look at the insides of the lips and mouth, and at the inner sides of the lower eyelids. These places are a nice, healthy pink colour in a healthy person, regardless of his race. After heavy blood loss these places become pale, whether the person is coloured or not; the skin still feels cold and clammy and there is also a rapid, thready pulse.

2. *The pulse*

The pulse is really the impulse of a column of blood passing through an artery following the expulsion of blood from the heart during its contraction. The pulse most commonly felt for is the radial pulse. To feel your own radial pulse hold your right palm upwards. Now place the palm of your left hand against the back of your right lower forearm, just above the wrist, and then let your left fingers curl round onto the front of the lower end of your right radius (the forearm bone on the same side as the thumb). By exerting gentle pressure with your left fingers, you should be able to feel your right radial pulse with your left index, middle and ring fingers. If you now press down hard on the artery with your left ring finger, you will stop the blood flowing any further along the artery, and you will no longer feel the pulse with your left index and middle fingers. You will still feel it with your ring finger as the heart tries to pump blood past the obstruction. In other words, you have been able to compress the artery because it is soft and elastic (i.e. healthy). In old people, this is

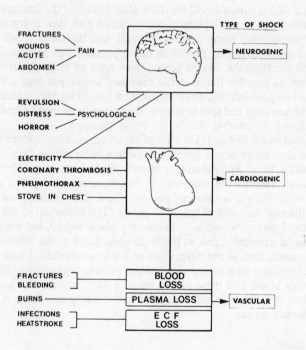

Fig. 6

often not possible to do, because the arteries become dilated and hardened during the ageing process. The radial pulse is the one most commonly felt for, but there are other places where arterial pulses can be felt – the Femoral pulse in the groin, the Carotid pulse in the neck and the Superficial Temporal pulse just in front of the ear. Anaesthetists find the superficial temporal pulse very convenient to use because they usually sit at the head-end of the operating table.

We feel at the pulse in order to determine its *Rate, Rhythm* and *Volume. The pulse rate* is the number of beats per minute, which can be determined with the aid of a watch with a seconds finger. The normal rate varies considerably. The resting pulse rate may be anywhere between

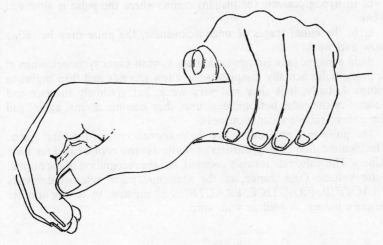

Fig. 7 Taking the pulse.

fifty and ninety beats per minute. *The pulse rhythm* is normally regular, even after injury. Irregularities can occur in heart disease, which does not usually concern the First Aider. What we mean by *the pulse volume* is the strength of the pulse. The normal volume of the radial pulse can be learned by feeling your own (as described above). You will also note that the femoral pulse has a greater volume than the radial pulse. This is because it is a bigger artery. For the same reason, the carotid pulse volume is greater than that of the radial artery, whilst the smaller, superficial temporal artery has a smaller pulse volume than any of the other three arteries mentioned.

Exercise (physical work, running, jumping, etc.) causes a normal increase in pulse volume and rate, because the heart has to pump out more blood per beat and at more beats per minute, in order to try to keep up with the body's increased energy consumption.

Abnormal increase in pulse volume occurs:

a. in the later stages of brain compression, after head injury.

b. in diabetic (ketotic) coma.

c. during the adrenaline response to injury.

d. in *acute* infections.

Please note, at this stage, that 'acute' means 'of rapid onset', and that 'chronic' means 'prolonged'. For example, tuberculosis is usually a chronic (prolonged) illness, whereas pneumonia is usually an acute illness (of rapid onset).

Abnormal reduction of pulse volume occurs:

a. typically after blood loss, when the pulse rate is increased, giving a typical *rapid, thready pulse*, together with a cold, clammy skin.

b. in hypoglycaemic (or insulin) coma, where the pulse is slow and weak.

c. in the initial stages of unconsciousness, the pulse may be rather slow and weak.

d. in a simple faint (otherwise known as vaso-vagal syncope), when at first, the pulse actually disappears for a few seconds and then begins to return. Initially, it is slow and very weak, but gradually the rate and volume of the pulse both increase until they become normal again, and the patient recovers consciousness.

The pulse *rate* and *volume* are the main concerns of the First Aider. The identification of irregularities of rhythm is too complicated for First Aiders. The pulse rate is easily counted, but the recognition of the normal pulse volume (and, hence, of the abnormal pulse volume) demands PRACTICE, PRACTICE, PRACTICE. So practise, by feeling at other people's pulses, as well as your own.

3. *Respiration*

When considering respiration, we want to know its *rate* and *depth*. The normal, resting respiration is fairly shallow, and its rate is about 16–20 per minute. The rate and depth of respiration are both increased during exertion of any kind, of course, and this is normal. However, deep and fairly rapid respiration occurs, together with a rapid, bounding pulse (increased pulse volume) in diabetic coma, because the person in diabetic (ketotic) coma is trying desperately to breathe out the poisonous ketones, which have built up inside him, and which are the cause of his coma. On the other hand, someone who is in a coma caused by an overdose of insulin (hypoglycaemic coma) will display rather slow and shallow breathing, together with a slow, feeble pulse. Air hunger has already been mentioned (see 'Facial Appearance'). It is very deep, sighing respiration and it occurs because of gross loss of red blood cells (i.e. tremendous blood loss). Because there are few cells left in his circulation, the injured person has to make the fullest possible use of his lungs in order to try to satisfy his need for oxygen. Therefore, he inhales and exhales fully, all the time. Obviously, such a person will be very pale, because the tremendous blood loss has thrown him suddenly into a severely anaemic state, and he will die soon unless he is transfued with *blood*, (at this stage, blood substitutes and plasma are inadequate, because they cannot compensate for the loss of the red cells).

There are two other kinds of respiration which should be mentioned:

a. Stertorous respiration. This is a rapid, shallow and noisy respiration. It is seen in chest injuries and, sometimes in abdominal injuries.

b. Cheyne-Stokes respiration. This is 'Crescendo breathing', in which the breathing gradually builds up from a slow and shallow stage to a rapid and deep stage. Then it gradually returns to a slow and shallow stage, after which period of *apnoea* (i.e. 'no breathing') follows. The

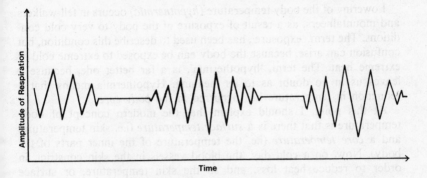

Fig. 8 Cheyne Stokes respiration.

pattern repeats itself, each crescendo being separated from the next by a period of apnoea.

When this Cheyne-Stokes form of respiration occurs, it is a sign that the person is near to death and beyond recovery – it is a *terminal sign*.

I have never known anyone survive once Cheyne-Stokes respiration has begun. It occurs commonly as a terminal sign in cases of head injury, although it could occur as a terminal sign in a case of diabetic (ketotic) coma.

Cheyne-Stokes respiration should not be confused with a type of respiration, which can occur in climbers in altitudes in excess of ten thousand feet above mean sea level. The climber may be breathing slowly and shallowly. Then suddenly, an outburst of deep, rapid respiration occurs, which tails off into slow, shallow respiration again within a few seconds. This type of high-altitude respiration should not be confused with Cheyne-Stokes respiration, because there is no gradual build-up of respiration to the deep, rapid stage. High-altitude respiration is the price, which Man pays for trying to exist at an altitude for which he is not designed.

4. *Temperature*

The temperature of the human body can be measured by using an oral thermometer, which can be placed into the mouth, or into the armpit. The most accurate reading is made by using a rectal thermometer. Special electronic rectal thermometers are now available, and they give a very accurate reading within seconds, where the usual mercury clinical thermometers take two or three minutes to give an accurate reading.

The normal *maximum* human body temperature is 37°C (98.6°F), but many normal, healthy people have temperatures of 36.1°C (97°F). The temperature of the body may be raised *slightly* after exertion, but any gross elevation of temperature occurs because of infection, heat stroke, or in the later stages of brain compression after injury.

Lowering of the body temperature (*hypothermia*) occurs in fell-walkers and mountaineers, as a result of exposure of the body to very cold conditions. The term, 'exposure', has been used to describe this condition, but confusion can arise, because the body can be exposed to extreme cold or extreme heat. The term, 'hypothermia', is a far better one, because it leaves us in no doubt as to its meaning. Hypothermia means that a reduction in temperature has occurred in the *body core*.

At this point, I should explain that the modern concept of body temperature is that there is a *surface temperature* (i.e. skin temperature) and a *core temperature* (i.e. the temperature of the inner parts of the body). Now, on a cold day, the blood vessels in the skin constrict, in order to reduce heat loss, and so the skin temperature, or surface temperature is reduced. This is no great detriment, as long as the temperature of the inner body, the core temperature, remains at a healthy level. However, once a person's core temperature begins to fall, that person has begun to suffer from hypothermia. Special rectal thermometers, which give readings to well below those obtainable with the ordinary clinical thermometers, are necessary to measure the body core temperature. Ordinary clinical thermometers are quite inadequate for this purpose.

5. Blood Pressure

I have made mention already of blood pressure in Part I, and of the fact that exercise causes an increase in the systolic blood pressure, but little, if any, increase in the diastolic blood pressure. In fact, it may cause a *decrease* in the diastolic blood pressure. It can be seen, therefore, that exercise must increase the pulse pressure. The pulse pressure is also increased by the adrenaline response. A fall in blood pressure is usually the result of heavy blood loss, when it is associated with a rapid, thready pulse; but it also occurs in the final stages of brain compression (just before death) and in insulin coma. In each of these cases, the pulse will become progressively slower and weaker.

Measurement of blood pressure

The instrument which measures blood pressure is a sphygmomanometer, or 'sphyg' for short. There are two kinds of 'sphyg':

a. *The mercury sphyg.* This shows the blood pressure by means of a column of mercury, in the same way as a mercury barometer shows atmospheric pressure.

b. *The anaeroid sphyg.* This functions basically like an anaeroid barometer. Anaeroid means 'without air'. The anaeroid sphyg is much lighter and more compact than the mercury sphyg, but it should be checked regularly against a mercury sphyg to be sure that it still reads accurately. If its accuracy decreases, it can be re-calibrated.

I shall now describe how to use a sphygmomanometer. First of all,

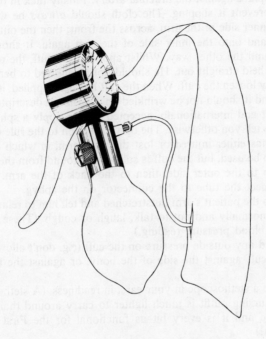

Fig. 9 Anaeroid sphygmomanometer and cuff.

there is a rather long piece of cloth which is to be wrapped around the right arm half way between the shoulder and the elbow. In one end of this cloth there is an inflatable cuff, and from this cuff either one or two rubber tubes emerge through the cloth (one or two tubes depending on who manufactured the sphyg and when). The tube, or tubes, will eventually be connected to the sphyg itself. The sphyg has a dial and below the dial there is a nut which, when tightened up, will prevent air from escaping. When loosened it allows air to escape. Below the nut there is a rubber bulb which, when squeezed repeatedly, pumps air into the sphyg system.

Method (The internationally accepted method)

1. Bare the *RIGHT* arm of the patient, and make sure there is no constricting object (e.g. a tightly rolled-up sleeve) which could cause a false blood pressure reading.

2. Squeeze all air out of the inflatable cuff.

3. Place the inflatable cuff on the inner side of the arm (over the

brachial artery) half way between shoulder and elbow. Wrap the rest of the cloth round and round the arm so that it keeps the cuff firmly, but not tightly, in place against the brachial artery. Finally tuck in the end of the cloth to prevent it slipping. The cloth should *always* be wound round from the inner side of the arm, across the front; then the outer side, then the back and onto the inner side of the arm again. It should *never* be wound round the other way. Whilst applying the cuff, the patient's arm should be held straight out. He should not be allowed to bend the elbow as this may loosen the cuff. When the cuff has been applied, it should be a snug fit, and it should not be wrinkled up. The above description is that of the correct and internationally accepted way to apply a sphyg cuff, and let nobody tell you otherwise. The only exception to the rule occurs when someone has either injured or lost the right arm, in which case the left arm has to be used, but the cuff is still wound round from the inner to the front, then to the outer side, then to the back of the arm.

4. Connect the tube to the connector on the sphyg.

5. Keep the patient's arm outstretched and tell him to relax his fingers, to breath normally and not to talk, laugh or cough. (These actions can affect the blood pressure reading.)

6. Avoid any outside pressure on the cuff (e.g. don't allow the arm to press the cuff against the side of the body, or against the bed or your knee).

7. Place a stethoscope in your ears, in readiness. (A stethoscope from a child's nursing outfit is much lighter to carry around than a doctor's stethoscope and it is every bit as functional for the First Aider's requirements!)

8. Place the index and middle fingers of your *left* hand flatly across the inner side of the front of the patient's *right* elbow (this is where his brachial artery crosses his elbow).

9. Pump the sphyg bulb repeatedly and rapidly until the needle points to about 100 mm. You should now be able to feel his brachial artery pulsing away under your left index and middle fingers. *Keep your fingers there*! Do not lose that spot! Now, carry on pumping until the brachial pulse can no longer be felt. The pressure in the cuff is now greater than the patient's systolic blood pressure (the upper blood pressure reading) because it is preventing blood from getting through to the forearm.

10. Now allow air to escape *SLOWLY*, by releasing the nut very slightly, and keep a sharp eye on the pointer. Note the reading on the sphyg when you feel the pulse return. This is the systolic blood pressure and this is the only way to find it – i.e. by feeling with your left index and middle fingers. You must NEVER listen for the systolic blood pressure before feeling for it. If you do listen, you *may* get away with it a few times, but eventually you will hear sounds which will lead you to record a falsely high, or falsely low systolic blood pressure.

11. Having found the systolic blood pressure (by *feeling* for it) apply the chest piece of the stethoscope to the place where you felt the brachial

pulse, and you will hear a 'Thump, thump, thump' as the blood passes through the artery. Keep the stethoscope there, and slowly release more air. The reading will fall, of course. When you hear a slight change in the force of the 'thump', note the reading. This is the diastolic pressure, and at about 5 mm below this reading, the 'thumps' should disappear altogether.

A word of caution here. You should watch the pointer on the dial and keep on listening until the pointer reads zero. The reason for this is that in some people (notably middle-aged men with somewhat raised blood pressures) the 'thump' sound appears at the systolic pressure, persists as the pressure reduces, then suddenly disappears, only to reappear later quite strongly, and then disappears later, just after the diastolic pressure has been reached, as described above.

The description of the steps to be taken may make the whole process seem to be a long one, but in fact, with practice, you will find that you can take a blood pressure in two minutes flat, or even less. Just one other thing I should mention and that is, that the blood pressure as recorded by one person may differ slightly from the blood pressure as recorded by another person. The reason for this is that we all have slightly different hearing abilities. For this reason, it is generally agreed that we record both systolic and diastolic pressures *TO THE NEAREST 5 mm* and therefore, your reading should not differ by more than 5 mm from anybody else's reading. You can practise taking blood pressure on each other.

Now that we have considered the foregoing indicators of the patient's general condition, we may proceed to the search for injuries.

The search for injuries

The examination has begun already by assessing the temperature, pulse, respiration, blood pressure and facial appearance. Apart from facial appearance, simple observation can reveal some 'give-away' attitudes. For example, in the case of a fractured clavicle, the patient typically inclines his head towards the injured side and hugs the shoulder of the injured side with the hand of the uninjured side.

In the case of a dislocated shoulder, the normal, rounded appearance of the Deltoid muscle (the muscle covering the upper, outer third of the humerus) can no longer be seen, and instead the Deltoid muscle is flattened out by comparison with the normal side. The injured side is supported below the elbow by the hand of the normal side, whilst the elbow of the injured side is semi-flexed. When the elbow is dislocated, there is loss of the normal bony triangle (this will be mentioned again, when I deal with injuries to bones and joints). The dislocated elbow is held semi-flexed and the limb is supported, just above the wrist, by the hand of the normal side. A similar attitude is adopted when there is a supracondylar fracture of the humerus. In Colles' fracture, as every First Aider knows, there is a typical 'dinner fork' deformity. In young children, a condition called 'pulled elbow' may occur, (to be described in *Injuries to Bones and Joints*) and in this condition the whole of the upper limb hangs limply, because it is too painful for the child to lift that limb.

The 'give-away' attitudes of the lower limbs are, of course, those of the hip injuries. In fractured neck of femur (*NOT* impacted fracture of the neck of the femur), there is typically a shortening of the injured limb with the foot everted (turned outwards). In dislocation, or fracture-dislocation of the hip, the injured hip is held in flexion, internal rotation and adduction (pulled towards the midline), and the knee is therefore, held in flexion, so that the foot can support the weight of the limb.

So far, we have used our powers of observation (Inspection), but now we get round to feeling (Palpation). The patient may say that his thigh hurts, and there may be an obvious deformity of the femur. He may say he has pain in his leg, and there may be an obvious deformity of the tibia and fibula. Nevertheless, it is still important to feel for injuries, for the following three reasons, which are very basic but very important:

1. *Pain* is a purely personal sensation, and it is a *symptom*. A symptom is something of which the patient complains. Pain should not be confused with *tenderness*, which is a *sign* – i.e. something elicited on examination. Tenderness means that when we exert pressure over an injured area we cause pain. It is common to have a complaint of pain at a certain site and to be able to elicit tenderness at that site. However, it can happen that tenderness may be elicited at a site where the patient did not complain of pain.

2. Furthermore, if a patient has two injuries, he may be so distracted by the pain from the first site of injury that he does not complain of pain at the second site of injury. In such a case, the second site of injury is said to be '*masked*' by the pain from the first site.

3. A person may be injured in one place, and yet the pain of that injury may be felt in another place. This is known as 'referred pain'. The prize example of referred pain occurs when a person with a fractured neck of femur complains of pain in the knee on the same side (fractured neck of right femur, pain in right knee), but not of pain in the hip.

This phenomenon of referred pain can be explained by Hilton's Law. Hilton was an anatomist. He found that when a muscle acts upon a joint to alter the position of that joint, then both the muscle and the joint receive nerve fibres from the same nerve. The muscle receives motor nerve fibres to make it contract, and the joint receives sensory nerve fibres, which carry sensory impulses to the brain. These sensory impulses inform the brain of the joint's position, (whether the joint is flexed or extended). Now, the Quadriceps muscle on the front of the thigh helps to flex the hip and also to extend the knee, whilst the Hamstring muscles at the back of the thigh, help to extend the hip and to flex the knee. So, we have two groups of muscles, each acting on the same two joints. Therefore, using Hilton's Law, we can see how easy it is for the brain to confuse the two joints after injury. In fact, the brain is interpreting the pain as coming from the knee, when really the injury is in the region of the hip joint.

For the three reasons just stated, it is clear that every patient MUST be examined from head to toe, so that sites of *tenderness* will not be missed. With practice, you should be able to go over a patient from head to toe in two minutes.

Method

Always examine from the patient's right side, unless you are left-handed in which case it is permissible to place yourself to the left of the patient.

A certain amount of pressure must be applied with *flat* fingers to all parts of the head, and the limbs must be squeezed firmly all down their length in order to find tenderness. To give yourself a good idea of the correct amount of pressure to be exerted, place your fingers flat on the top of your head and press downwards until you can feel a definite pressure build up in the back of your neck. That is the correct amount of pressure to use when pressing or squeezing. It will elicit tenderness without causing damage. The exception to this rule occurs when a person is unconscious and *MAY* have a depressed fracture of the skull. In the unconscious patient, the scalp and skull-vault must be palpated *VERY GENTLY*, in order to find swellings or depressions only. The unconscious patient cannot tell you that you are causing pain, and there is no sense in adding to any depression already present in the skull-vault.

For the purpose of the following exercise, I will assume that the patient is conscious. Initially, as you practise on each other, you will find it beneficial to assume that consciousness exists. Most injured people are conscious when found, anyway.

1. *Head and neck.* Face the patient, and firstly, feel gently over the skull vault for lumps or depressions and for lacerations of the scalp. All of these can be missed if we simply look. They must be felt for. Even blood is not easy to see in the hair, especially if the hair is dark. Blood is sticky and will be transferred to your fingers and be seen.

Next, press firmly (as described previously) over *all* the skull vault, including the forehead, temples, mastoid bones (behind the ears) and the occiput (the lower part of the back of the skull). Use both hands at the same time and look for bleeding or CSF from the ears whilst you are feeling. Clotted blood should be wiped away from the ear. This helps to distinguish between bleeding from inside the ear and blood which has trickled into the ear from a scalp wound. Then press down onto the nose (unless it is obviously deformed and bleeding). After this, press on each cheek bone simultaneously and continue pressing along the *zygomatic arch* (the bony arch or ridge which passes from the cheek bone to just in front of the ear). When you reach the front of the ear, move downwards, one fingerwidth only. One finger of your right hand should now be on the patient's left jaw-bone-joint, and one finger of your left hand should be on his right jaw-bone-joint. These joints are called the temporomandibular joints, or TM joints for brevity. (Thank Goodness for abbreviations!) Now, ask the patient to move his jaw up and down and then from side to side. In each case you should feel the normal, smooth movement occurring in the TM joints. Any rough movement, or 'crunching' feeling in these joints is abnormal. Now feel firmly down the jawbone right to the point of the chin, for deformity, swelling or loss of normal contour, tenderness and, possibly, crepitus (see *Injuries to Bones and Joints*). Remember to look inside the mouth for lacerations to tongue or cheeks, broken or loose teeth, and for blood trickling down the back of the throat which would indicate bleeding from behind the nose. If the person has had a head injury, it is worthwhile taking note of the pupils at this stage (see *Head injury*).

Lastly we examine the neck. Press firmly on the vertebrae of the cervical spine, working downwards from the base of the skull. *If no tenderness is found*, check the neck movements. Tell him to put his chin onto his chest (i.e. full flexion), then to put his head right back (i.e. full extension). Now, tell him to turn his head *fully* to the left and then *fully* to the right (i.e. full lateral rotation to left and right). Finally, tell him to make his left ear touch his left shoulder and then to make his right ear touch his right shoulder (i.e. full lateral flexion of the neck to left and right). Note any restriction of movement. If tenderness is found initially, do *not* check the movements. Splint the neck forthwith. That completes your examination of the head and neck.

2. *Upper limbs*. Press with the flat fingers over the collar bones and shoulder blades. Next, squeeze the limbs, with the same amount of pressure, all the way down from the shoulder right to the fingers. Squeeze both upper limbs at the same time. Note any sites of tenderness, which will be re-examined later in more detail, (described in *Injuries to Bones and Joints*). If no tenderness is found, complete the examination of the upper limbs by ensuring that the joints all pass through a full range of movements. If tenderness is found in one upper limb, complete the examination of the *uninjured* limb.

Testing for joint movements in the upper limb
  a. Shoulder. The basic movements at this joint are:
    i. Flexion – i.e. raising the arm forwards, to point directly upwards.
    ii. Extension – i.e. the exact opposite of flexion.
    iii. Abduction – i.e. raising the arm sideways, away from the body.
    iv. Adduction – i.e. the exact opposite of abduction.
    v. Internal rotation – i.e. rotating the humerus, so that the front of the elbow comes to face inwards, towards the body.
    vi. External rotation – i.e. the exact opposite of internal rotation.
Tell the patient to place his hands behind his back, with his fingers

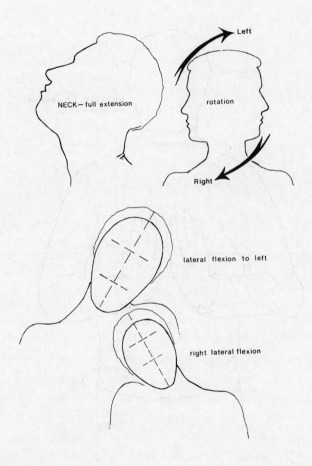

Fig. 10 Neck movements.

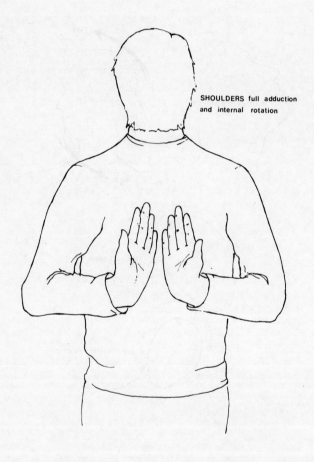

SHOULDERS full adduction
and internal rotation

Fig. 11 Shoulder movements.

BONY TRIANGLE OF ELBOW

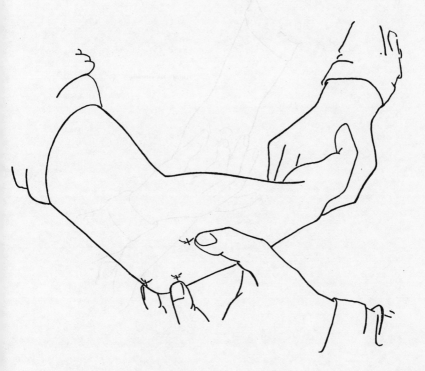

Fig. 12 The bony triangle of the elbow.

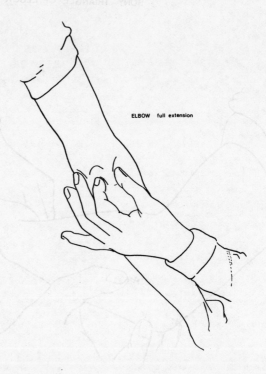

ELBOW   full extension

Fig. 13 The bony triangle becomes a straight line (elbow fully extended).

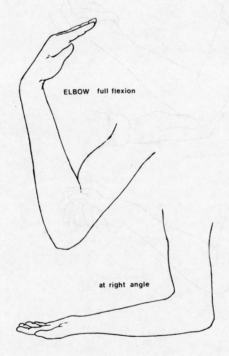

Fig. 14 Elbow movements.

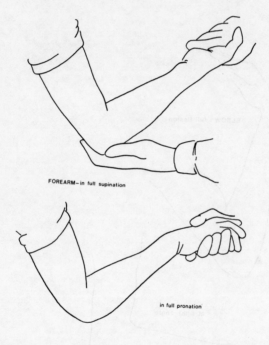

FOREARM – in full supination

in full pronation

Fig. 15 Forearm movements (Note the 'hand-shaking' technique).

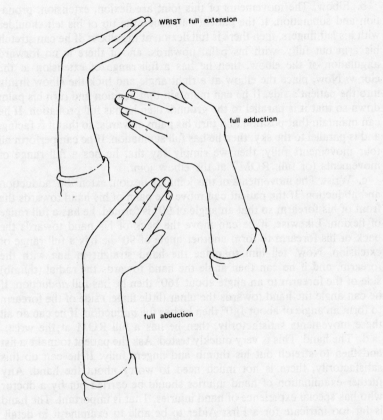

WRIST full extension

full adduction

full abduction

Fig. 16 Wrist movements.

pointing up his spine (this is full extension, internal rotation and adduction combined). Then, tell him to place his hands behind his head and to push his elbows right back (this is full abduction and external rotation, combined). Finally, tell him to raise his *straight* arms above his head and place the palms of his hands together (this is full extension). If he can perform all of these movements, then he has a full range of movements in the shoulders.

b. Elbow. The movements of this joint are flexion, extension, pronation and supination. If the patient can touch the tip of his left shoulder with his left fingers, then there is full flexion at the elbow. If he can stretch his arm out fully, with his palm upwards, and if there is no forward angulation of the elbow, then he has a full range of extension at the elbow. Now, place the elbow at a right angle and tuck the elbow firmly into the patient's side. If he can maintain that position and turn his palm down so that it is parallel to the ground, then he has full pronation. If he can maintain that position and turn his palm upwards, so that it is facing, and is parallel to the sky, then he has full supination. If he can perform all four movements fully, then we simply say that he has a full range of movements (or full 'ROM') at the elbow joint.

c. Wrist. The movements of this joint are flexion, extension, adduction and abduction. If the patient can move the palm of his hand towards the front of his forearm so that an angle of 90° is formed, he has a full range of flexion. Likewise, if he can move the back of his hand towards the back of his forearm to form another angle of 90° he has a full range of extension. Now, tell him to place the hand straight in line with the forearm, and if he can then angle the hand towards the radial (thumb) side of the forearm to an angle about 160° then he has full *ab*duction. If he can angle the hand towards the ulnar (little finger) side of the forearm to form an angle of about 140° then he has full *ad*duction. If he can do all these movements satisfactorily, then he has a full ROM at the wrist.

d. The hand. This is very quickly tested. Ask the patient to make a fist and then to stretch out his thumb and fingers fully. If he can do this satisfactorily, there is not much need to worry about the hand. Any further examination of hand injuries should be carried out by a doctor who has special experience of hand injuries. That is important. The hand is far too intricate for a First Aider to be able to examine it in detail. *ALWAYS* refer hand injuries for a medical opinion, no matter how trivial the injury may seem to be.

3. *The chest.* The idea is to 'spring' the ribs by quickly compressing and releasing them. Place one hand on the left side of the rib cage and your other hand on the right side, below the armpits. Quickly compress the chest, by pressing your hands towards each other and release immediately. Note whether the patient winces or catches his breath. Now, place one hand over the sternum and the other over the dorsal (thoracic) spine. Repeat the 'springing' procedure and again note if the patient winces or catches his breath.

N.B. If the patient is a young lady, then the hand to be used on the sternum should be used as a 'clenched fist' and the soft part of the fist (the little finger side) should be the part to be placed on the sternum, because knuckles hurt. I advise you to use a clenched fist in this way, because placing a flat hand upon the front of a young lady's chest may cause her to think that your intentions are not entirely honourable!

4. *Spine and sacrum.* (a) Preferably, the patient should be asked to sit up for this (but see (b) below). With the patient sitting and leaning forwards, use the soft part of the fist to hump fairly heavily all down the dorsal (thoracic) spine, lumbar spine and over the Sacrum. Do not worry, you will not do any harm, and you will soon elicit any tenderness. (b) If the patient cannot sit up then you will have to slide your left hand underneath the patient. Having done this, keep your fingers straight and press upwards with the tips of the fingers onto the spine. Repeat the process down the whole length of the spine. A left-hander is allowed to do this with his right hand. If you are using this method correctly, then you should be able to 'lift' the patient slightly every time you press upwards.

5. *Hips and pelvis.* Find the pubic bone (the bone at the 'pit' of the abdomen) and press on it. Follow the extensions of this bone as they pass towards the left and right groins, pressing on them, too. If no tenderness is found, place your right hand a few inches above the patient's left hip joint. You should feel the crest of the left hip bone. Do the same with your left hand above his right hip joint and find the crest of the right hip bone. Now, try to squeeze the two hip bones together between your hands. If any pain is caused, ask the patient to point to it. Now, slide forwards along the crest of each hip bone, until you feel it take a sharp downward turn. With the 'heel' of each thumb, press backwards on both of these downward-sloping parts of each hip bone simultaneously. Again note the site of any pain. You have just compressed the pelvis from side to side and from front to back, just as you compressed the chest in two directions.

Hips. Press over the front of each groin and then move sideways until you come to the greater trochanter (the upper end of the femur). Thump both right and left greater trochanters with the soft part of the fist. Note any tenderness.

6. *Lower limbs.* You have begun the examination of these by thumping the hips. Now, quickly squeeze down the whole length of each lower limb (as you did with the arms) and note any sites of tenderness. If no tenderness is found, check the range of movements of the joints.

For the purposes of this exercise, let us assume that no tenderness has been found in the lower limbs. This means that we now have to check all the joints of the lower limbs for a full range of movements. Now, in order to test the ROM of the hip joint, the whole of the lower limb has to be moved. So, having squeezed your way down the lower limb to the toes, let us now work our way upwards again, through the joints of the lower

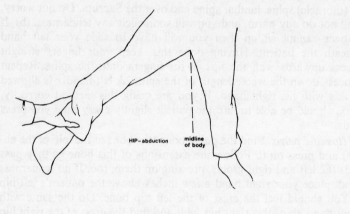

Fig. 17 Abduction of the hip.

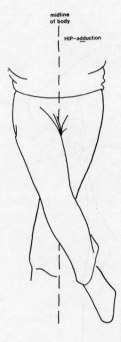

midline
of body

HIP—adduction

Fig. 18 Adduction of the hip.

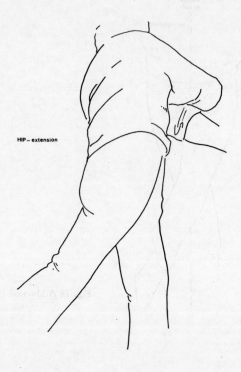

Fig. 19 Extension of the hip.

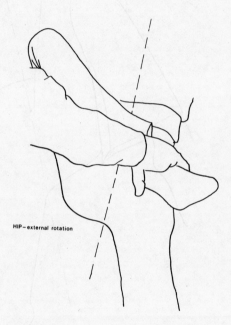

HIP – external rotation

Fig. 20 External rotation of the hip (knee faces outwards).

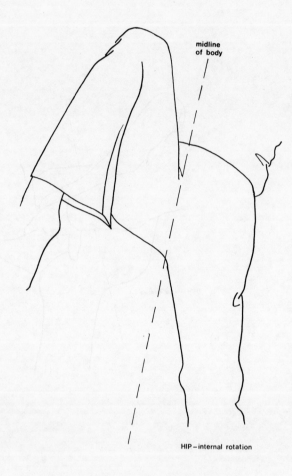

midline
of body

HIP—internal rotation

Fig. 21 Internal rotation of the hip (knee faces inwards).

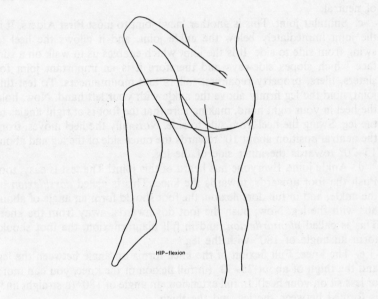

HIP-flexion

Fig. 22 Flexion of the hip.

limbs.

a. Toes. Simply push them all up together and then push them all down together. This is merely to see if there is any restriction of movement in one toe compared with the others.

b. Mid-tarsal joint. This is a 'new' joint as far as most First Aiders are concerned. Quite simply, it is a joint formed amongst the bones of the tarsus and allows a small amount of rotation of the forefoot upon the hindfoot. To test this joint, hold the heel firmly in your left hand and then take hold of the forefoot, across the metatarsals, with your right hand. Now, twist the forefoot from side to side, trying to keep the heel fixed. You should find a range of movements which is about 5–10° either side of neutral.

c. Subtalar joint. This is another 'new' joint to most First Aiders. It is the joint immediately below the ankle joint, and it allows the heel to swing from side to side. It is the joint which enables us to walk on a surface which slopes sideways and therefore it is an important joint for slaters, tilers, property repairers, sailors and mountaineers. To test this joint, hold the leg firmly above the ankle with your left hand. Now, hold the heel in your right hand, making sure that the foot is at right angles to the leg. Swing the heel from side to side. Normally the heel moves, from the neutral position about 10° towards the outer side of the leg and about 15–20° towards the inner side of the leg.

d. Ankle joint. Everyone has heard of this joint! The test is easy, too. Push the foot upwards, towards the knee. This is called *dorsiflexion* of the ankle, and in full dorsiflexion, the foot should form an angle of about 80° with the leg. Now, push the foot downwards, away from the knee. This is called *plantarflexion*, and in full plantarflexion, the foot should form an angle of 180° with the leg.

e. The knee. Full flexion of the knee forms an angle between the leg and the thigh of about 25–30° (in full flexion of the knee, you can more or less sit on your heel). In full extension, an angle of 180° (a straight line) is formed between the leg and the thigh.

Approach the knee as follows:

i. Look and feel for swellings in or around the knee.

ii. Ask the patient to lift the heel off the ground and hold the knee straight. If he can do this, then:

iii. Say, 'Keep your knee straight and do *not* let me bend it.'

iv. Now, try to bend his knee. If the quadriceps muscle, at the front of the thigh is of normal strength, and if the patella is not damaged, you will not be able to bend his knee.

v. With the knee in the same fully extended position, try to bend it to either side. If the ligaments on either side are intact, the knee will not bend from side to side.

vi. Finally, tell the patient to relax and see if the knee flexes (bends) fully.

If a First Aider can drill himself to examine a knee as well as that, then

I shall be amply satisfied. It would be very unfair to ask a First Aider to examine a knee in any greater detail than I have described above. The examination for cartilage injuries is a difficult art which takes years of practice and experience to learn.

f. The hip. There are six movements which occur at this joint. They are:

i. flexion – movement of the knee up towards the chest. Normally, the knee can touch the chest.

ii. extension – the opposite direction. From the standing position, the thigh can normally swing backwards through about 30–40°.

iii. abduction – movement of the lower limb away from the midline of the body. The normal maximum range of abduction is about 45°. Very supple people can achieve a much greater range than this (e.g. those who can do the 'splits').

iv. adduction – movement of the lower limb towards and across the midline of the body. In other words, 'crossing one's legs'. The normal maximum range of adduction is about 35–40°.

v. internal rotation. If you stand with your knees absolutely straight and then turn your feet inwards, you will find that your knee-caps are also facing inwards. Now, the amount of rotation which can occur at the knee and ankle is very slight indeed. Therefore, the movement must have occurred mainly at the hip. The normal maximum amount of internal rotation is 40°.

vi. external rotation. This is turning the feet outwards. The normal maximum external rotation is 60°.

vii. *Straight-leg raising*. Before I go on to describe the examination of the hip joint, I should explain that there is a *test for compression of the spinal cord* (e.g. by a 'slipped disc'). This is called the *Straight-leg Raising test* (SLR for short). The straight leg is simply raised as far as it will go. The leg will normally go far enough to form a right angle with the rest of the body. The test is carried out with each leg separately. Make allowances for people with tight hamstring muscles (not enough exercise!) because they complain of tightness behind the knee, when the leg has been raised through about 80°. However, if there is any cord compression, then there will be limitation of SLR and the patient will complain of sudden pain in the lumbar spine at the same time as the limitation of SLR becomes apparent. If this happens, note the angle to which the limb was raisable, (e.g. 70°, 60° or 30°) and *RECORD IT*. (30° would represent gross restriction of straight-leg raising.)

The examination for hip movements

a. Carry out SLR as described above. Note any limitation or lumber pain.

b. Bend the knee and continue to bend the hip till the knee touches the chest.

c. Bring the hip back to form a right angle with the body and, keeping the knee at a right angle also, swing the foot outwards, away from the midline. This is INTERNAL rotation of the hip joint. Note the angle which the leg (i.e. tibia) forms with the midline of the body.

d. Now, swing the foot in the opposite direction (across the midline). This is EXTERNAL rotation of the hip joint (the knee-cap points outwards). Note the angle which the leg forms with the midline of the body.

e. Put the first leg down straight and repeat (a) to (d) with the second leg.

f. Finally turn the patient onto the left side, place your left hand firmly on his pelvis, and pull each leg backwards in turn (the patient should be facing away from you now, if you are examining him from his right side, because you have turned him onto his left side). Note any restriction of extension. *N.B.* If you feel the patient's pelvis move, then you have reached the limit of extension of his hip.

7. *The abdomen.* This is the next in line for examination. I will not burden you with the details at this stage, because I have given you enough to be practising already. For the time being, once you have com-

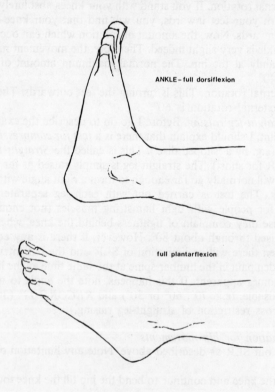

ANKLE – full dorsiflexion

full plantarflexion

Fig. 23 Ankle movements.

pleted the skeletal examination, just place a hand on the abdomen and say, 'Abdomen', so that you will train yourself not to forget! The examination of the abdomen will be dealt with in 'Abdominal Injuries'.

8. *The chest* (again!). I know that we have already been there, but it may be necessary to take a closer look. More detailed examination of the chest is discussed in 'Chest Injuries'. For the time being, just put a hand on it and say 'Possibly chest'.

The foregoing description of head-to-toe examination may seem to be very long-winded indeed. If it does, then the reason is probably that most, or all, of the procedures mentioned are new to you. However, once you start to put the scheme into practice, you will find that each part of it takes far less time to do than to read, and eventually, your aim should be to cover the bones and joints in two minutes flat. Practise on each other. In fact you can practise most of the joint movements on yourself.

The advantage of this scheme is that you will not be fooled by referred pain, masked pain or absent pain. You will not be deceived into accepting the patient's word that he has 'no injury', or that he has 'only hurt his arm'. By using this scheme you will find whatever injuries are to be found. You will also satisfy yourself that the rest of the body is intact and that *there are no more injuries to be found*. With this comforting reassurance in mind, you can confidently devote your attention to treating the injuries found. In the case of mass casualties, you can confidently assess your patients' order of priority of evacuation. So, *please* learn the system of head-to-toe examination thoroughly, and it will serve you well.

Before passing on to Part III, let us summarise what we have done so far.

Summary of Parts I and II

In Part I, the normal function of the body was described. Much of Part I was necessarily factual. Facts are facts, and sometimes they have to be learned by sheer, hard slogging. There is no other way.

In Part II we developed the scheme of taking the history, assessing the general condition of the patient and examining the patient. I also mentioned a number of pitfalls to be avoided (e.g. NEVER simply accept the patient's word that he is 'alright'. ALWAYS satisfy yourself that he is all right).

Now it may not always be essential to take the blood pressure, or to record the temperature, or even to count the rate of respiration. It is essential ALWAYS to feel and assess the pulse. This is good medicine.

So, let us recapitulate on the scheme we have developed.

The scheme (condensed)
1. Approach the patient with calm reassurance.
2. Start to take the history and, whilst the patient is answering you feel

and assess the pulse and take a good look at his face (not so closely that you force him to ask what you are looking at!)

3. Look for any 'give-away' attitudes.

4. Go through the system of head-to-toe examination.

5. Take the temperature, respiratory rate and blood pressure, where necessary.

Apart from developing the above scheme in your mind, I have given you (I hope) a great deal of food for thought. I have tried to give you the benefit of my experience in Part II, so it is up to you to take advantage of it.

In addition, I have described how to take a blood pressure and how to examine the whole of the skeletal system. I trust that you will practise these techniques regularly and as often as possible. In between your practice sessions, you can browse through Part III, *Specific Subjects*.

PART III: Specific Subjects

Introductory note

These specific subjects are those with which I dealt during a series of talks to the Rossendale Fell Rescue Team. At the end of the talks, I asked the team to take a test which I had prepared for them, and eighteen members of the team obliged. Now, the talks had lasted a total of ten to twelve hours. The object of the test was to find out just how well the team members had absorbed this concentrated bombardment of information. The test was mostly factual, but a few parts of it required ingenuity. The results were even better than expected. This made me think that if they could do so well in such a short time, then surely people elsewhere should be able to learn just as well, *provided* they could read the same information in their own good time, with each learning at his or her own individual rate of learning.

I shall deal with the subjects in the same order as when I talked to the Rossendale Fell Rescue Team.

Depending upon your previous knowledge, you may be covering 'old ground' as you read through these subjects. Nevertheless, I hope that you will find them interesting.

A final topic which has been added onto this list of Specific Subjects is entitled, 'Mass Casualties'. I hope that this will be of some benefit to search and rescue teams.

CAUSES OF UNCONSCIOUSNESS (AND DIAGNOSIS OF DEATH)

There are quite a few possible causes of unconsciousness, and an apparently unconscious person may, in fact, be dead. Fortunately, there is an easy way to remember the common causes of unconsciousness. All you have to say to yourself is 'A,E,I,O,U and 3 Ds'.

Our scheme for remembering the causes of unconsciousness can now be written out as follows:

'A' — Apoplexy (i.e. Stroke)
Asphyxia.

'E' — Epilepsy (and Epileptiform convulsions, especially in children)
Embolism — i.e. massive pulmonary embolism (usually fatal)
Exposure — either to extreme cold or to extreme heat (heat stroke)

Electric shock.

'I'   — Injury — i.e. Head injury

Infarct — i.e. Myocardial infarct or Coronary thrombosis, or Heart attack

Simple faint — Sorry, this is an 'Odd one in'!

'O'   — Overdose.

'U'   — Uraemia, gross kidney malfunction.

'3 Ds':

Diabetes — hyperglycaemic or hypoglycaemic coma

Drunk — alcoholic intoxication

Dead.

I do not claim to be the originator of this scheme. It has been used for a long time. It is not one hundred per cent complete, because there are tropical diseases, such as malaria, which can cause unconsciousness and a few rare conditions which the First Aider is most unlikely to see, but this list gives the common causes of unconsciousness, which the First Aider may well encounter. Let us now go over our scheme in rather more detail:

'A'

1. *Apoplexy* or Stroke is caused by either a *cerebral haemorrhage* (i.e. bleeding into the brain tissue from a blood vessel) or a *cerebral thrombosis* (i.e. a blood clot blocking an artery in the brain tissue). In both of these conditions, the onset is usually quite sudden, and it usually leads to a complete paralysis of one side of the body — i.e. face, upper limb and lower limb. Because of weakness of the cheek on the affected side of the face, there is a typical 'blowing' sound as the patient exhales. The eyes often look towards the affected side of the brain (i.e. *away* from the affected side of the body) and the speech area may be affected (see '*Nervous System*' in Part I). The patient is typically elderly and may be conscious or unconscious.

Three other conditions which can be included under the heading of Apoplexy are Subarachnoid haemorrhage, Meningitis and Encephalitis. All three can result in unconsciousness.

2. *Subarachnoid haemorrhage* occurs typically in young men in springtime. A *sudden* bleed takes place from the arterial system which surrounds the base of the brain; therefore the onset is sudden. A typical history would be, 'He was bending down to tie his shoe laces, when he suddenly fell to the floor unconscious'. The breathing is often deep and may be stertorous (noisy). The limbs are often rigid, but may be flaccid. The pupils are sometimes unequal and show a tendency to vary in size independently of each other. However the typical finding is *neck rigidity*. If you place your hand behind his head and try to bend his neck so that his chin touches his chest, you will not be able to do so. You may even lift him half way into a sitting position but you will not be able to bend his neck. This is *true* neck rigidity. *It is a sign of irritation of the meninges*

(the coverings of the brain and the spinal cord). In this case, it is caused by the bleeding which has occurred *outside* the brain tissue, but *inside* the meninges.

3. *Meningitis and encephalitis* occur typically in children, though any age-group may be affected. From the First Aider's point of view the two are indistinguishable. The onset takes place over a few days. The child complains of feeling unwell, may complain of a sore throat and becomes lethargic. A temperature develops and increases until the child looks flushed and feels very hot when you feel at his forehead, and he is very likely to be vomiting at this stage. Again, the typical finding is neck *ridigity* which, in this case, is caused by inflammation of the meninges by the infection. *N.B.* Do not mistake *meningism for neck ridigity*. Meningism occurs quite commonly in such conditions as influenza. The patient complains that his neck feels stiff, but his neck can be bent forward and his chin can be placed upon his chest though it may cause him a little discomfort.

When feeling at the forehead to see if it feels hot use the skin on the backs of the middle bones of your fingers. This skin has better temperature appreciation than the skin on any other part of the hand.

When meningitis is well advanced, the patient may arch his back spontaneously. This is called Opisthotonos and it may be so severe that the patient may be arched upwards, supported only by his head and heels.

4. *Asphyxia* is caused by anything which prevents the normal exchange of oxygen and carbon dioxide in the lungs. The causes can be divided into physical and chemical. The *physical causes* include such things as smothering, strangulation and inhaled foreign body — i.e. anything which physically prevents the air from passing into or out of the lungs. The *chemical causes* include poisoning by gases such as carbon monoxide and hydrogen cyanide (Prussic acid). These chemicals are able to combine very strongly with the haemoglobin in the red cells, and having done so, they block the ability of haemoglobin to combine with either oxygen or carbon dioxide. The result of this is that the body suffers from lack of oxygen. *The treatment* of asphyxia is to remove any physical cause, give mouth-to-mouth resuscitation where necessary, and to remove the patient to hospital, especially when poisonous gas is suspected to have caused the asphyxia.

'E'

1. *Epilepsy* is a condition characterised by intermittent convulsions. It is *not* familial. The commonest cause is brain damage at birth, though there are quite a number of possible causes, e.g. when epilepsy occurs for the first time during adult life, it is usually as the result of a severe head injury. *Very occasionally* it may be the first sign of a brain tumour. Please note that I said 'very occasionally'. So, do not go around diagnosing brain tumours right, left and centre!

The typical sequence of an epileptic attack begins with the Aura, followed by the Tonic phase, the Clonic phase and Flaccid phase, in that order. *The aura* is the warning phase, which often lasts only 15–30 seconds. During this phase, the patient knows he is going to have a fit, but he cannot warn anyone. Those who know the patient well may notice a certain vague appearance on his face and can prepare for the convulsion.

The tonic phase occurs suddenly. The patient falls to the ground and all his muscles tense up; he becomes completely rigid, not even breathing. He may become blue in the face (cyanosed), because this stage may last half to one minute. His face usually assumes a grimace.

The clonic phase occurs next. All the muscles of the body twitch violently, repeatedly and independently of each other. This may last up to two minutes, and it is during this phase that he froths at the mouth. He may pass urine and even faeces, because he has lost voluntary control of his bladder and bowels.

The flaccid phase takes over from the clonic phase. He relaxes, breathes more normally, though maybe heavily at first, and appears to be asleep. His colour returns to normal. This stage *may* last ten minutes or even more, though it may be over within a minute.

N.B. (a) *Automatism* may occur sometimes after an epileptic fit. This is a state in which the patient appears to have returned to normal, but he performs automatic actions, e.g. going for a bus ride. This state may last for up to twenty-four hours. For obvious reasons, an epileptic must not be left alone for twenty-four hours after a fit. (b) *Status epilepticus* is a condition where one fit occurs and before the patient has fully recovered from it, another one begins and this is followed by another, etc. It is a series of fits strung together. If this occurs, you must get the patient to hospital or he will die.

2. *Epileptiform convulsions.* These commonly occur in children, but could occur in adults. A very high temperature causes spontaneous triggering-off of the nervous impulses in the brain and the result is a convulsion, which may be followed by more convulsions. The most effective first-aid measure is to tepid-sponge the patient *all over*, to bring down the temperature. If the temperature is brought down and *kept down*, the convulsions will stop.

3. *Embolism.* An embolus is a blood-clot, which commonly forms in a vein of a lower limb or in a vein in the pelvis. When the clot breaks free, it can travel along in the bloodstream towards the heart. A very small embolus will pass through the right atrium and right ventricle and will lodge finally in a lung. A *massive* pulmonary embolus will lodge in the pulmonary artery. Thus, it will stop the flow of blood through the lungs and the victim suffers from lack of oxygen. Therefore, he collapses suddenly, becomes cyanosed and unconscious and will be very fortunate if he survives. So get him to hospital immediately!

4. *Exposure*

    a. *To extreme cold.* I have already mentioned this in Part I. I will remind you that a special rectal thermometer is necessary to register temperatures below 95°F (35°C). It is useful to be able to detect hypothermia in its early stages, because the sooner it is detected the better for all concerned. So, if you are out on the hills in a group, be on the lookout for any member of the group who may start to look rather cold, unhappy and perhaps pale. If you *suspect* early hypothermia in anyone, then first of all take off a glove and leave your hand exposed for 10–15 minutes, so that your hand becomes cold. Now apply the temperature-sensitive part of your fingers to his cheeks and forehead (see *Meningitis*), and if his face feels cold to your already cold fingers, then he has already begun to suffer from hypothermia. If the appropriate treatment is commenced at once, he will probably recover well enough to walk off the hill, under escort. If his condition is allowed to deteriorate, undoubtedly he will have to be carried off, eventually. A little astute observation can prevent a lot of trouble.

Hypothermia also occurs in the elderly. It occurs commonly in those who live alone. They are usually elderly widows, because women have a longer life-span than men. Either she falls in the house, fractures the neck of the femur and is unable to attract anyone's attention; or she becomes too old and too frail even to feed herself, and one day she finds she is too weak to get out of bed; or she may be confined to bed by an illness (e.g. pneumonia or a stroke). In any case, it may be a day or more before anyone finds her and during this time her body cools because the fire goes out, she is immobile and she cannot increase her slow metabolic rate enough to maintain a healthy body temperature.

The treatment of hypothermia is aimed at restoring the body core temperature to normal. To this end, it is essential to remove wet clothing and to prevent further heat loss. The exact method of rewarming has been a moot point for some time. Rapid re-warming, by immersion in a hot bath, has been advocated as a treatment for hypothermia in the younger age-groups. In my opinion, this method of treatment is fraught with the danger of circulatory collapse and death. Rapid re-warming definitely kills old people.

Gradual re-warming is the method of choice in both young and old. The elderly are usually taken to hospital, where they are allowed to warm up gradually in bed. No hot water bottles are used. Young people suffering from hypothermia are usually found on a mountain or a hillside. *It can be positively harmful* to place a person suffering from severe hypothermia onto a stretcher and then race down the mountain in order to get him to hospital as soon as possible. The rough ride will cause a marked deterioration in his general condition. *The treatment of choice* for such a person is to pitch a tent (if possible), place him inside it, make sure that he is well-insulated from the ground, remove all wet clothing, cover him up and use one or two other people to act as 'human hot water bottles'. I call this the 'Eskimo treatment', because the Eskimos have used it successfully for hundreds of years.

The victim of hypothermia, treated this way, can be re-warmed in the safety of shelter and knowing that he is no longer alone. It may take twenty-four hours for him to regain a normal body temperature, but when he has done so, and when he has rested and eaten, he should be able to walk down the mountain, under escort. So, do not be in too great a hurry to get him off the mountain. Patience, in this case, brings its own rewards.

b. *To extreme heat (Heat stroke).* If a person's heat-losing mechanisms fail (i.e. sweating, vasodilation and panting) then he will complain of a headache, become extremely weak and flushed and eventually he will lose consciousness; his temperature will soar upwards and he will die. He should be protected from the heat source, tepid-sponged, or (if necessary) placed in an ice bath.

5. *Electric shock* may cause unconsciousness (see 'infarct' below).

'I'

1. *Injury to the head* is dealt with later (see *Head Injuries*)

2. *Infarct (or coronary thrombosis).* In this condition the patient complains typically of a severe tight or crushing pain in the front of the chest and there may also be pain down the left arm, or even down both arms. Occasionally there may be pain in the front of the neck, but this is far more common in angina. The pain is so severe that the patient is often pale and sweating, and he may vomit. He may collapse and become unconscious because of heart failure. Sometimes, a person who suffers a massive coronary thrombosis may just collapse and become unconscious, without even complaining of pain. External cardiac massage has been advocated in the past but on more than one occasion it has done the patient more harm than good.

In one case, a woman who collapsed was treated with external cardiac massage, but died. A post mortem examination revealed fractured ribs, lacerations to the liver and a rupture of the diaphragm, with gross bleeding into the abdomen, which was considered to be the cause of death. The moral from this is 'Either do it right, or just do not do it'. I, myself, have tried to revive people by cardiac massage (external *and internal*), when they have collapsed after coronaries. So far, my failure rate is 100 per cent! In other words, external cardiac massage is most unlikely to restart a heart which has stopped because of a coronary. It is far more likely to be successful after electric shock, but even then, another electric shock from a defibrillator is far more likely to be successful. The reason for this is that, after an electric shock the heart muscle itself is not damaged, but it has lost its ability to contract in a properly co-ordinated fashion. A coronary thrombosis causes the death of a part of the heart muscle, and therefore the dead part of the heart muscle is unable to contract, no matter what you do to it.

Those people who are revived by external cardiac massage after a coronary thrombosis are usually found to have had a small infarct, which has affected the heart's ability to contract in a co-ordinated fashion (cf. electric shock). The most important thing is to confirm the diagnosis of cardiac arrest, *before* embarking upon external cardiac massage. The diagnosis is confirmed by:

a. inability to feel a pulse, and

b. inability to hear a heartbeat.

If external cardiac massage has been continued for ten minutes, and if the pulse cannot be felt, nor the heartbeat heard, then further cardiac massage will prove useless.

3. *Simple faint* (the high class name for this is Vasovagal syncope).

As I was saying, the simple faint usually occurs in a hot, humid atmosphere (typically, a crowded, poorly-ventilated room). The victim of the simple faint begins to feel weak and dizzy , starts to breathe slowly and deeply and his face becomes very pale as the blood pressure collapses and then, losing consciousness (because blood is not reaching the brain), he falls to the floor. Now, a word of caution at this point. This picture can easily be mistaken for that of a collapse following a coronary thrombosis. So, first of all allow the patient to lie flat on his back, raise the feet about one foot (30 cm) above the ground, loosen the clothing around the neck and then feel at the pulse. At first, in a simple faint, the pulse and heartbeat disappear, because the blood is pooled in the lower parts of the body and no blood is returning to the heart. Once the person is lying on the floor, the blood can flow horizontally back towards the heart, which then begins to pump blood around the circulation again. This is Nature's way of dealing with a simple faint, and it is the best way. As you feel for the radial pulse, you will feel it returning, very slowly and weakly at first, but gradually and steadily, the pulse rate and volume increase, until they are back to normal and the person regains consciousness. By raising the feet you will speed recovery by making it easier for blood to return to the heart. Until the blood returns to the heart, the person will remain unconscious, because blood and oxygen are not reaching the brain. Therefore, I will stress the following two points:

a. The person suffering from a simple faint should *ALWAYS* be allowed to lie down. You must *NEVER* prop him up against a wall or in a corner. This in turn, prolongs the brain's oxygen-lack, and *you could kill him this way*!

b. Before you dive headlong into performing external cardiac massage, *PLEASE BE SURE* that the person is not merely suffering from a simple faint!

'O'

Overdose. Opiates are the derivatives of opium, which comes from the opium poppy. They include Morphine, Pethidine, Codeine, Papaveretum, ('Omnopon') and Diamorphine ('Heroin'). Nowadays, there are many other drugs which, in overdose, can cause unconsciousness. These newer drugs are members of the two groups known as Tranquillisers and Antidepressants and they are too numerous to list here (apart from which, I would not wish to incur the wrath of any particular drug firm!) There is also the group of drugs known as Barbiturates. These have been on the market for many years.

A person who has taken an overdose of a drug first of all becomes drowsy but rouseable. Later he becomes unrouseable but irritable. Then he becomes unresponsive, and during this stage the pupils vary in size individually. At one moment the right pupil may be larger than the left, and the next moment the reverse may be the case. Depending on how much of the drug has been absorbed into the bloodstream, the person may die, or he may survive. If he survives, he will wake up with an almighty 'hangover'!

'U'

Uraemia. This is a condition in which there is a great build-up of urea in the blood. It occurs because the kidneys are so badly diseased that they are unable to perform their normal function. If a person is so uraemic that he becomes unconscious, then the outlook is very grave indeed. As a First Aider you are most unlikely to see this condition, because the patient will probably have been ill in bed for a long time.

'3Ds'

1. *Diabetes mellitus.* This should be no stranger to anyone, these days. I will simply remind you that there are two types of coma, which may occur in diabetes: (a) Hypoglycaemia (Insulin coma). It is caused either by not eating after a normal dose of insulin, or by an accidental overdose of insulin and it results in a low blood sugar. The patient becomes pale, cold and clammy, and his pulse becomes increasingly slower and weaker. If you reach him before he becomes unconscious, try to give him something to eat, preferably sugar or glucose. If he is unconscious already, he should be taken to hospital, because he needs to have glucose injected into a vein. (b) Hyperglycaemia (Ketotic coma). In this condition, the diabetes is out of control and the blood sugar is very high, hence the name *hyper*glycaemia (Hyper = above. Hypo = below). However, I must stress that it is NOT the increased blood sugar which is responsible for the coma. It is the build-up of ketones which does the damage. In diabetes mellitus, the patient cannot complete the breakdown of glucose into carbon dioxide and water. Instead, he reaches only the half-way stage in the breakdown process. He manages to break down each glucose molecule into two ketone molecules and is then unable to proceed any further. Since he has obtained much less energy from one glucose molecule than the normal person would, he continues his quest for further energy by liberating into his bloodstream far more glucose than the normal person would, and again the glucose is broken down only as far as the ketone stage, which is as far as the diabetic can go. Now, these ketones are poisonous to the human body. So, if they can be broken down into the relatively harmless carbon dioxide and water – as happens

in the normal person – then all is well. However, the diabetic *cannot* break them down. Instead he builds up a concentration within himself until a very dangerous level is reached, at which stage he goes into coma. If he is not treated promptly, he will die. So remember, it is the ketones which do the damage, not the glucose. For this reason *hyperglycaemic coma* is often referred to as *ketotic coma*.

The person in ketotic coma has a dry, flushed face, a rapid, bounding pulse and deep, rapid respiration. The sweet-smelling breath is due to the ketones, which he is trying desperately to exhale, just as a normal person would exhale carbon dioxide. He must be admitted to hospital so that:

    a. his life can be saved and,

    b. his treatment can be stabilised before he is allowed to go home.

If you compare the signs of hypoglycaemic coma and ketotic coma, you will see that the facial appearances are different, pulse rate and volume are different and so are the respiratory rate and volume. Therefore, normally, you should have little difficulty in distinguishing one from the other.

However, if you find a diabetic who is drowsy (i.e. in a pre-comatose condition) and if there is any doubt in your mind at all as to which kind of coma he is going into, then *make him eat sugar*, as much as possible. As I have said already sugar, or glucose, does no harm. Therefore, if he is going into hypoglycaemic coma, the sugar will revive him. If he is going into ketotic coma, sugar will not revive him, though it will do him no harm. This is the way to prove your diagnosis, one way or the other, and perhaps to revive the patient. So, NEVER BE AFRAID TO GIVE SUGAR TO A DIABETIC.

2. *Drunk* (i.e. alcohol intoxication). This speaks for itself! Since alcohol is a drug of intoxication it could have been included under Overdose, but it just happens to be convenient to use as the second of the '3 Ds'. Otherwise there would only be 2 Ds.

The signs are very similar to those of the overdose. Alcohol first causes a slight slowing of mental processes. Then it produces elation and the person appears more alert, and may increase the speed of speech, writing etc. However, at the same time, the *accuracy* (of speech, writing, driving, typing etc.) is *decreased*. Later, speech and actions become progressively slower, and unconsciousness supervenes. The 'give-away' sign is, of course, the smell of alcohol on the breath. Having said that, it should be pointed out that a drunken man may collapse because of a stroke, coronary thrombosis, epilepsy, etc.

3. *Dead* (and *diagnosis of death*). Death is death, or is it? Death can be defined in many ways, none of which is complete and accurate in itself. When a person has ceased to be capable of functioning as an independent individual, the cells of the body continue to function for a number of hours afterwards, until each cell, in its own time, gradually grinds to a halt. Therefore, death is extremely difficult, if not impossible, to define. It is much easier to accept that death is death and that we know of certain

signs, which enable us to make a diagnosis of death. I know that death is a diagnosis which First Aiders are reluctant to make. Perhaps this is because it is so final, and they do not wish to declare someone dead, who may be alive. However, it is important to be able to make this diagnosis, especially when dealing with mass casualties, when priority of evacuation becomes so vital. Those in the worst condition must be evacuated first, if you are to save the maximum number of lives possible. Obviously you would not send a dead person to a mortuary in preference to sending a living person to hospital. Also, you would send a conscious person with multiple injuries away first, in preference to an unconscious person already displaying Cheyne-Stokes respiration, whose chances are nil. The ethics of priority of evacuation in peacetime are debatable, but the object should be to save as many recoverable people as possible and not to en-danger the recoverable lives by giving priority of evacuation to the irrecoverable. Let us now consider the signs which assist us to make the diagnosis of death.

a. *Early signs of death.* If you come across a dead man soon after death then usually you will find that he is motionless, but on occasions, there may be spontaneous unco-ordinated twitching movements, es-pecially if death has been caused by violent crush-injury to the head. These movements last for only a few minutes. Electric shock may cause an immediate stiffening of all the muscles of the body, known as Cadaveric Spasm. Usually however, the limbs are found to be quite flac-cid (i.e. floppy). The eyes are fixed and staring, with the pupils fixed, dilated and unresponsive to light. Both the lash reflex and the corneal reflex are absent (see notes 1 and 2 below). The pulses are absent (radial, carotid and femoral), as is the heartbeat. Chest movement is absent and the 'mirror-sign' is negative (see note 3). If you place your ear to his chest, you will not hear any breath sounds, but be careful not to press on the chest, or you may expel air and this would give you the false impres-sion that he is alive! About twenty minutes after the circulation has ceas-ed, the corneae (the 'windows' of the eyes) become glazed and opaque. This is because of lack of lubrication of the corneae by tears, which have ceased to be produced by the tear glands.

Explanatory notes

1. *Lash reflex*
   If you touch your own, or someone else's eyelash, it causes the eyelids to blink. This is the lash reflex.

2. *Corneal reflex*
   CAREFUL! This is very painful to the conscious person. If you touch the cornea it will cause a sustained blink. Just think of the last time someone poked a finger into your eye!

3. Mirror sign

If you hold a mirror, or other dry, shiny surface, near the mouth, then condensation settles onto that surface from the expired air. There is no condensation of course, if the patient is dead.

4. Heartbeat

How to find the apex beat is dealt with in 'Chest Injuries'.

b. *Later signs of death*. From the First Aider's point of view, these are: Asphyxia Livida, Asphyxia Pallida and Rigor Mortis. I shall not discuss the effects of decomposition, because I hope that you will never have to come across the gruesome remains of anybody, weeks or months after death.

For the purposes of this description let us assume that the dead man is lying on his back.

Asphyxia pallida is a pallor of the parts of the body furthest away from the ground. In this case, that would be the face, and the front of the trunk, arms and legs. It is caused by the effect of gravity, which causes the blood in the skin to move slowly towards the ground.

Asphyxia livida occurs for the same reason. The blood which, in this case, has flowed towards the back of the head, neck, trunk, arms and legs, causes those parts of the body to have a purplish, mottled appearance, except for the parts actually in contact with the ground – i.e. the pressure points, which are actually bearing the weight of the body.

The above two processes are both part of the same gravity effect, and therefore they occur together, at the same rate. The gravity effect starts as soon as the circulation has ceased and asphyxia livida and asphyxia pallida are usually noticeable within a couple of hours.

Rigor mortis. I mentioned before that once circulation has stopped, the individual cells of the body continue to use energy until they gradually die. The muscle cells are no exception to the rule. Since the blood is no longer bringing an oxygen supply to the muscles, they have to break down their glucose supply by a very slow process. This causes the onset of a very slow contraction of the muscles, which eventually passes off when there is no further source of energy left. This process is called rigor mortis.

It is a chemical process, and chemical processes are speeded up by increasing the temperature and they are slowed down by decreasing the temperature. Thus, the speed at which rigor mortis takes place is influenced by the temperature of the environment in which the body is found. It occurs much faster in babies than in adults, because babies have a higher metabolic rate than adults.

Generally in adults in temperate climates, rigor commences at about three hours after death with stiffening of the muscles of the face, extends to the arms, hands and feet, and eventually, at about *twelve hours* after death, the whole of the body is involved in a generalised stiffness. The stiffness, or rigor, is then said to be fully established and it remains so for a further *twelve hours*. It gradually passes off during the next *twelve hours*, and from then on the body remains flaccid. The whole process of rigor is completed thirty-six hours after death.

In jungle conditions, the time taken to complete the process may be only eighteen hours, and in babies, even in temperate climates, it may be completed in nine hours.

A note of the state of rigor mortis when a body is found, and a note of the time when rigor passes off, can be *legally* important, for many reasons, and can help to establish the time of death.

It should be noted that Scottish law is different from the law of England and Wales. This has always been so, and the laws relating to death are no exception to the rule. In Scotland, a dead body must be seen by a doctor as soon after death as possible. This is absolutely essential in Scottish law, but it is not necessarily so according to the law of England and Wales.

Nevertheless, as I have stated previously, it is important to be able to recognise death. This is particularly important when dealing with a number of injured people. Those, who are alive and who can be restored to health, MUST be evacuated in preference to the dead. The dead must be evacuated last of all. Since there may be no doctor at the scene of the accident, the decision must be taken by the people on the spot.

HEAD INJURIES

'To explore, or not to explore the cranium?' That is the question. The decision to operate on someone who is suffering from a head injury is made by doctors in hospital. Their decision is based on the history of the injury, the findings on examination, and by observation of the progress of the injured person. This observation is carried out for twelve hours after the head injury, whether the person is conscious or not, because the first twelve hours after a head injury is the danger period, during which compression of the brain (by bleeding inside the skull) can occur. If it is more than twelve hours after the head injury, and if the patient is fully conscious, head injury observation can be discontinued.

Now the doctor can examine the patient and see the injuries for himself, but he often has to rely upon other people for the history of the injury, and neither a doctor nor a nurse in hospital can commence observation of the patient until he has reached hospital. The sooner the observation commences the better it is for patient, doctor and nurse. For example, let us suppose that a man is injured on a mountain. He is unconscious when found and because evacuation is difficult, it takes three hours to get him to hospital. If observation is begun only after he reaches hospital, then we have lost the first three recordable hours of the patient's progress. If observation begins when he is found, we have those first three hours on record and this gives us a far more complete picture of the patient's progress. The picture during those first three hours may be the factor which persuades the doctor whether to operate or not. It is especially important, too, when you bear in mind the fact that it may take an hour or two to get a rescue team up the mountain to him in the first place. *So, here is a real chance for the First Aider to shine.*

The immediate First Aid treatment of any unconscious person must be to ensure that the airway is clear and to stop haemorrhage. In fact, these are the two First Aid actions which save life more than any others. You must *NOT* however, try to stop bleeding or CSF from the nose or ears, because to do so would pre-dispose to infection. Bacteria would have an easy access to the inside of the skull and an infection inside the skull is the *last* thing a head-injury victim needs! Having taken care of the immediate First Aid, we now deal with the situation as follows:

1. *History*
    The object here is to find out, as accurately as possible:
    a. the time of the injury,
    b. the duration of unconsciousness and
    c. the length of retrograde amnesia (I will explain what this means later).

Every scrap of information can be vital and should be recorded, no matter how irrelevant it may seem at the time. Therefore, not only should you question the injured person if he has regained consciousness, but you should question anybody who witnessed the accident, because the injured person may not even recall the accident at all. It is quite common for him to remember events up to a few minutes before the accident, but then he remembers nothing until a point in time after the accident. In other words, he has Amnesia, (loss of memory). If we can ascertain the time of his last memory recollection *before* the accident and the time of the accident itself, then we can calculate the time of *Retrograde Amnesia*, which is the length of time between his last memory and the accident.

For example, the man with the head injury says that he remembers setting off in the morning, and he remembers the moment at which he reached the top of Scafell Pike. He remembers nothing further until he woke up and found people standing around him. Let us say that, from the man himself, and from witnesses, we ascertain that the top of Scafell Pike was reached at 10.30 a.m. and that he woke up at 11.00 a.m. The total length of amnesia is 30 minutes. However, the witnesses tell us that he fell at 10.50 a.m. Therefore the duration of Retrograde Amnesia is from 10.30 a.m. to 10.50 a.m. – 20 minutes. (Retrograde means 'stepping backwards'. In this case going backwards in time from the accident.) The 10 minutes of amnesia *following* the injury (going forward in time from the accident) is known as anterograde amnesia.

Before we proceed any further. I owe you an explanation and a word of caution. Our brains perform many functions, one of which is memory-storage. Facts and events can be stored in the brain, just as they can in a computer. However, just as it takes time to programme a computer, so it takes a little time to store facts in the brain. The whole purpose of storing facts in our brains is to enable us to recall those facts for use at a later date. The most important facts are stored indefinitely (everyone knows his own date of birth), but the relatively unimportant facts are stored for only a very short time (e.g. most of us could not recall what we ate for lunch on 19th April, 1973, unless of course, it was a day to remember, such as a friend's wedding day!) A blow to the head can interfere with the memory storage process. This explains why the victim of a head injury cannot recall events for a certain length of time. He cannot recall events because his brain has *been unable to store them*. That is the explanation. The importance of assessing the length of retrograde amnesia as accurately as possible is that *the length of retrograde amnesia is directly proportional to the severity of the head injury*.

Now, let me caution you about the wily ways of *Anterograde Amnesia*. Let us take the same example but with a slight modification. The man remembers reaching the top of Scafell Pike at 10.30 a.m. and the witnesses confirm this. The witnesses maintain that he fell at 10.50 a.m. and that he woke up at 11.00 a.m. Furthermore the witnesses say that he was able to get up, he appeared perfectly normal, could speak and answer questions rationally, and he even walked back to base. Our man on the other hand, states quite categorically that he remembers nothing after reaching the top of Scafell Pike until they were arriving back at the base, which was at 11.30 a.m. What a peculiar conflict of stories! Is our man lying, or did everybody else mistake the time? In fact, nobody is mistaken. It is the same problem of inability to store memories in the injured brain. *The man's memory-storage function did not recover until 11.30 a.m.*, although he was conscious and rational from 11.00 a.m. In this case, therefore, we have anterograde amnesia of 40 minutes (i.e. from 10.50 a.m., when he was injured to 11.30 a.m.). This includes 10 minutes of unconsciousness. We also have the same 20 minutes of retrograde amnesia.

Anterograde amnesia is not very important from a First Aider's point of view, and you should not waste time trying to puzzle it out. I merely wanted to warn you that it can have puzzling effects. Your main aim, in taking the history is to assess as accurately as possible the three things I mentioned initially — i.e. the time of injury, the duration of unconsciousness and the length of retrograde amnesia. Once you have assessed these three things, write them down, concisely and *LEGIBLY*, e.g.:

'Time of injury = 10.50 a.m. Witnesses confirm this.'

'Unconsciousness = 10 minutes. Witnesses confirm this (woke up at 11.00 a.m.)'

'Retrograde amnesia = 20 minutes — Patient remembers top of Scafell Pike at 10.30 a.m.'

In these three lines you have covered the essential points of the history. If the patient has not recovered consciousness, you cannot assess the length of retrograde amnesia, because you cannot question him. You would then write:

Time of injury = 10.50 a.m. − witnesses confirm this.
Patient still unconscious at ... (time you reach him).

2. *Examination*

Having safeguarded the airway and arrested haemorrhage, approach the patient as described in Part II. Feel at the pulse and look at the face, whether he is conscious or not. If the signs of shock are present − pallor, cold, clammy skin and a rapid, thready pulse − then be on the look-out for other injuries, apart from the head injury, because shock is *not* usually a feature of head injury. When we use the word 'Shock' on its own, we are referring to the general condition of the patient which is produced by gross blood loss, stove-in chest injury, or a penetrating wound of the abdomen. Gross blood loss would be the result of external haemorrhage, or of bleeding internally into the abdomen or thorax (chest), or of blood loss from fractures. So, if you do find the signs of shock in someone with a head injury, *beware!* A certain amount of pallor of the face may be seen in someone who has just recovered from being unconscious, but the skin is not cold and clammy and there is no rapid, thready pulse. This pallor is due to concussion. *Concussion* simply means brain injury and the diagnosis of concussion can be made when a person, who has had a blow to the head, has retrograde amnesia. He usually has a headache too!

Let us proceed with the examination. Having felt at the pulse and looked at the face, we then look for bleeding and/or CSF from the nose and ears, and we feel for lacerations, depressions, haematomas and oedema. Lacerations are easily felt, so is the blood from them. Depressions in the skull are surprisingly difficult to feel. A *haematoma* is a collection of blood in soft tissues. It can occur anywhere, but in this context, a haematoma would lie between the skull and scalp. On pressing upon it with your fingers (as if you were playing a piano) it would feel crinkly, rather like a piece of soggy tissue paper. *Oedema* is a soft-tissue swelling caused by an increase of fluid amongst the cells in the soft tissue. The fluid does not form a pool, but is interspersed among the cells. If you come across this swelling and you press your finger into it for about five seconds, you will find that the pressure of your finger has left an indentation, or a 'pit mark'. This pitting is typical of oedema. If it is found on the scalp, it is virtually always indicative of a skull fracture and the fracture is usually directly underneath the oedema. In other words, *oedema of the scalp is virtually diagnostic of a skull fracture and it marks the fracture site.*

The rest of the examination should be carried out as described in Part II. Make a list of all injuries found, and indicate with drawings where any lacerations, haematomas or oedema of the scalp are found.

3. *Observation*

I have already explained the reason for this. For the sake of completeness, the nurses in hospital take the patient's blood pressure and temperature each time they observe the patient. Unfortunately it is not practical for a mountain rescue team to take the blood pressure and temperature every fifteen to thirty minutes during the evacuation of the patient, because he is firmly strapped down to a stretcher. If you wish, you may take the blood pressure and temperature when you examine the patient initially. The periodic observation which you will be able to carry out, during evacuation of the patient, will be of the other five factors, which are observed when the patient is under observation in hospital. These are: (1) Pulse, (2) Pupils, (3) Respiration, (4) Level of consciousness and (5) Level of response.

1. *The pulse.* Even though the patient may be strapped firmly to a stretcher, you can arrange it so that you are able to assess the patient's radial or carotid pulse. Remember, you want to record the rate, rhythm and volume of the pulse; e.g. '60/min regular, normal', or it may be '90/min irregular, feeble'. Accepted abbreviations are 'reg' for regular and 'irreg' for irregular.

2. *Pupils.* These should be observed for the following:

   a. Size – whether constricted, normal or dilated (e.g. Right dilated; Left normal).

   b. Reaction to light – brisk, normal, sluggish or absent. You should always check for the *Consensual light reflex*, too. To do this, shine a light into one eye and shield the other eye from the torchlight. The pupil of the eye into which the light is shone normally constricts. So, too, does the pupil of the other eye, even though the light is not shining into it. The second pupil is, in fact, constricting in sympathy with the first pupil. This is the consensual light reflex. So, your record might be: 'Reaction normal; Right and Left, consensual reflex normal'. *Please do not* write R for right and L for left. The *written* capitals R and L can be mistaken for each other. You may find this hard to believe, but it is true.

3. *Respiration.* We want to know the rate and type of respiration. The rate of respiration can be counted. The types are: normal, shallow, deep, stertorous (noisy) or Cheyne-Stokes. There could also be deep, sighing respiration as in air hunger. Your record of respiration, for example, might be, '23/min shallow'. In Cheyne-Stokes respiration which is crescendo breathing with periods of apnoea (no breathing) the rate of respiration varies, of course. Therefore, you simply record 'Cheyne-Stokes'.

4. *Level of consciousness.* Various diagrammatic methods of representing the level of consciousness have been devised, but they are not satisfactory. Let us take, for example, the method of shading in part of a square. One observer's *impression* of the state of consciousness of a patient may be to shade in a quarter of the square, whilst another observer's impression of the same patient's state of consciousness may be to fill in half a square. It is far better, therefore, to use a system of *words*, which we all understand. These words are:

1. Conscious.
2. Orientated (knows where he is and what is happening).
3. Disorientated (does not know where he is. He is confused).
4. Irritable ⎫
5. Drowsy ⎬   Self explanatory.
6. Rouseable (goes to sleep but can be awakened).
7. Unrouseable (asleep and cannot be awakened).

If you use these words, your record will be understood by hospital staff.

5. *Level of response.* Just as with level of consciousness, a system of words is by far the best means of recording the level of response. We record as follows:

Responds to:
1. Normal voice
2. Shouting
3. Tickling
4. Turning over
5. Pressure
6. Pain (e.g. nipping the skin)
7. Severe Pain (e.g. drive a knuckle firmly into the middle of your own breast bone. You will find it quite painful)
8. Unresponsive (i.e. does not respond to any of the above).

Again, by using this system of words, your record will be understood by hospital staff. That is very important for the continuity of the treatment of the patient, once he has reached hospital.

In conclusion, I would stress the following points:

1. Your history, examination and observation should follow the above scheme.

2. Your records should be legible. Other people have to read them!

3. Your observations should be carried out every fifteen minutes, if possible. Every thirty minutes is acceptable, especially if evacuation is long and difficult.

4. Finally, I would suggest that you contact the hospital in your area, so that you may see how the hospital head injury record sheet is printed. You can then arrange it so that the format of your head injury record corresponds to that of the hospital. This will eliminate another possible source of confusion. Some hospitals use charts which combine the records of head injury and multiple injuries, and this type of chart is known as a Major Accident Record.

I have already explained what is meant by concussion, but before I leave the subject of head injuries, I would like to clarify what is meant by *Compression.* A depressed fracture of the skull may exert a small amount of pressure on the brain, but this pressure does *not* continue to increase. However, when there is bleeding inside the skull, the blood cannot escape and it cannot expand the rigid skull vault. Therefore, the increasing pool of blood has no alternative but to extend inwards, inside the skull. This, in turn, causes a *continuous, progressive pressure on the brain* and this is what is meant by compression.

Let us consider the classical example of compression. This occurs as a rupture of the Middle Meningeal Artery, which is a small artery inside the skull, running along the inner surface of the temporal bone. The typical story is that the injured person received a blow to the temple. He may or may not have been unconscious. Either way, he seemed to have recovered well enough. Later, perhaps after a few hours, he complained of a headache, vomited and became drowsy. He would then gradually pass into unrouseable unconsciousness and unresponsiveness, and we would also see the pupils change. Depending upon whether the bleeding is occurring inside the right side or the left side of the skull, one side of the brain is compressed first, usually the side of the brain on the same side as the bleeding. (Occasionally, the opposite side of the brain is affected first). A typical sequence of pupil changes would be as follows:

Stage 1. Left pupil constricts (Right pupil still normal)
2. Right pupil constricts (Both now constricted)
3. Left pupil dilates (Right pupil still constricted)
4. Right pupil dilates (Both dilated).

When Stage 4 is reached, neither pupil will react to light, and the corneal reflex will soon disappear. The blood pressure, pulse rate and volume, and respiratory rate and volume will probably have all increased by this time, and all of them will soon fall fairly quickly to nothing. The patient may exhibit Cheyne-Stokes respiration before he dies. This is the classical picture of Compression. It is stressed because if the skull is explored in time, the bleeding can be stopped, the blood clot evacuated, and the patient can be restored dramatically to a normal state of physical and mental health.

INJURIES TO BONES AND JOINTS

The fractures which can occur in the various bones of the body, and how to deal with those fractures, are dealt with quite adequately in the First Aid Manuals. I will not waste your time by repeating a whole list of fractures. I will remind you of the 'give-away' signs and the 'head-to-toe' method of examination, which I described when discussing the search for injuries. I will remind you, also, that some fractures may be painless for a few hours after injury, because of the adrenaline response, that the patient may have referred pain, and that the pain of one fracture may mask the pain from another. These facts serve to emphasise the importance of *feeling* for tenderness and/or crepitus. The patient should be examined from head to toe. Any points of tenderness should be noted as you go along. When you have been over the patient from head to toe, you can then examine the tender places in more detail. I shall now deal with the cardinal signs of fracture, a few general points about joint injuries and the estimation of blood loss from fractures, in that order.

1. *The cardinal signs of fracture*

Nobody has X-ray eyes, and unless we come across somebody who has an open ('compound') fracture, we cannot actually see the broken bone. Closed ('simple') fractures are far more common than open fractures. Incidentally it is far better to use the terms 'Closed' and 'Open' than to use the terms 'Simple' or 'Compound'. The reason for this is that the word 'Simple', in everyday language, is the opposite of 'Complicated', and therefore, when talking of fractures, the terms 'Compound' and 'Complicated' can be confused. A *complicated* fracture is one in which there is damage to other structures (e.g. blood vessels and nerves) associated with the fracture, and a complicated fracture may be open or closed. So, please try to avoid the use of the words 'Simple' and 'Compound'.

Since the First Aider cannot take X-ray films, he has to rely on the five cardinal signs of fracture, which are:

a. Loss of function.

b. Deformity.

c. Abnormal mobility

d. *Localised* bony tenderness.

e. *Bony* crepitus (This is diagnostic of a fracture).

You may not find all five of these signs at the site of every fracture. However, if you find any two, or more, of these signs in combination at the site of injury, you can reasonably assume the presence of a fracture at that site, until proved otherwise by X-ray films.

Let us consider our five cardinal signs of fracture individually.

a. *Loss of function.* The patient may say that he cannot use his wrist, or hand. By your own observation, you may see that he cannot use them. If you ask him to squeeze your fingers, you will find that his grip is either very weak or even non-existent. He will say that it hurts him to even try to grip your finger. Why should this be so? Well, when a muscle acts upon a normal bone it does not cause pain because the bone is intact. When a muscle acts upon a fractured bone, it tends to cause movement at the fracture site, and any movement at the fracture site causes pain. Therefore, the patient declines to use the injured limb, rather than suffer the pain. Also, the fracture has upset the normal mechanics of the limb.

b. *Deformity.* This may occur as a result of the initial injury, or as a result of muscle spasm after the injury. The deformity itself may be a combination of any of the four different types of deformity, which are:

i. Angulation – i.e. one fragment forms an abnormal angle with the other.

ii. Rotation – i.e. one fragment may twist in relation to the other.

iii. Displacement – i.e. one fragment is moved sideways in relation to the other.

iv. Shortening – i.e. the fragments override each other, causing a shortening of (say) one femur compared with the other. The shortening is actually caused by spasm of the thigh muscles. This muscle spasm oc-

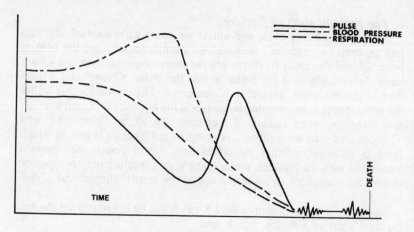

Fig. 24 Typical progressive changes in pulse rate, blood pressure, and respiratory rate during the late stages of the brain compression.

curs reflexly after injury, and it tends to reduce movement (and therefore pain) at the fracture site.

c. *Abnormal mobility.* This explains itself. If movement occurs where it should not, e.g. in the middle of the tibia and fibula – this is abnormal mobility.

d. *Localised bony tenderness. Localised* is the key word here. Generalised bony tenderness may occur if a bone is bruised. Tenderness localised to one particular point of the bone should make you suspicious of a fracture. It is worth noting, too, that where a bone lies just under the skin (e.g. skull, tibia, ulna and clavicle) there may be *oedema* at the fracture site. (Oedema was referred to in 'Head Injuries').

e. *Bony crepitus.* This is a rather unpleasant crunching sound, caused by any movement which results in the grating together of the fragments of the broken bone. Apart from being an unpleasant sound, bony crepitus causes the patient considerable pain. For this reason you should never search for it deliberately. If you do hear it, or feel it, then it is diagnostic of a fracture. I emphasise the term 'bony crepitus' because there is also soft-tissue crepitus, which is quite different and which will be referred to when we consider 'Chest Injuries'.

These then, are the five cardinal signs of fracture, and you should remember them, because (apart from the 'give-away' signs) they are the only guides which the First Aider can rely on when trying to rule out fracture, or to make a diagnosis of fracture.

2. *Joint injuries*

Swellings in joints caused by injury cannot be diagnosed accurately without X-ray films. Therefore, it would be grossly unfair to expect a

First Aider to make an accurate diagnosis of a swollen joint. So, if a joint is swollen, simply splint it and take the patient to hospital. Before going further, I will caution you *against* trying to manipulate a dislocation, or fracture-dislocation. The ability to manipulate successfully and *safely* depends on two things. Firstly, the manipulator must have an inborn knack for manipulation and this is composed of three things:

  a. the ability to use *controlled* strength to a very fine degree;
  b. a *very* sensitive touch;
  c. the ability to hold a mental picture of what is happening to a joint, as he manipulates it.

Secondly, the manipulator must have been through a course of *training*. So, the general rule for First Aiders is NOT to manipulate joints. However, having said that, I think you should be aware of the injuries which can occur to joints, because it will make you more aware of the need for X-ray films before a diagnosis can be made. I will list the injuries first, and then discuss them. The injuries are:

  1. Sprain.
  2. Contusion (internal bruising).
  3. Internal derangement.
  4. Fracture into a joint.
  5. Dislocation.
  6. Fracture-dislocation.
  7. Pulled elbow (in children).

After many joint injuries, a fluid swelling occurs in the joint. The joint swells up and if you squeeze *gently* your fingers can feel the fluid fluctuate under their pressure. This fluid swelling is called an *Effusion*, and an effusion, after injury, may be composed of:

  a. synovial fluid;
  b. blood, or
  c. a mixture of both.

The history can give us a good idea of what kind of effusion it is. If the patient says that the joint had swollen up within fifteen to twenty minutes, then it is 'odds-on' that the effusion is blood. If the swelling occurred, say, up to an hour after the injury, the effusion is probably a mixture of blood and synovial fluid. If it took longer than an hour for the swelling to develop, then that effusion is highly likely to be composed of synovial fluid alone. These effusions are seen quite frequently in the knee, ankle, elbow, wrist and finger joints. Now, let us discuss the injuries.

1. *A sprain* is an injury which causes stretching of the capsule and the synovial membrane of a joint. The synovial membrane responds to the injury by pouring out excessive synovial fluid, to form an effusion. If there is a small tear in the synovial membrane, the fluid will contain some blood. (*N.B.* the word *Strain* should not be used to describe a joint injury. A strain is a stretching injury of a tendon or muscle.)

2. *A contusion* is a form of internal bruising, caused by a jolting injury to the joint. The jolting blow causes temporary damage to the articular car-

tilage which covers each bone end. As a result of this, the articular cartilages lose their ability to move against each other smoothly, and any attempted movement causes pain. In order to try to compensate for this, the synovial membrane pours out much more of the lubricating synovial fluid than usual, the object being that the fluid should separate the articular cartilages, restore smooth movement and ease pain. So much fluid is needed to do this, however, that the effusion bulges the joint capsule, and this in itself causes aching. Overall, the general effect of the effusion is a reduction of pain caused by the contusion. Contusion of the elbow and knee are quite common.

3. *A fracture into a joint* causes an effusion of blood into that joint, because the fracture-line has breached the articular cartilage, and the way is clear for blood to flow from the fracture-site into the joint. The joints commonly involved in this kind of injury are the elbow, the knee and the ankle. The swelling of the joint occurs within fifteen to twenty minutes after the injury. The lesson to be learned here is that, *if you have reason to believe that an effusion has been caused by bleeding into a joint, then it is reasonable to suspect a fracture involving that joint, until you are proved wrong by X-rays.*

4. *Internal derangements.* I have put this in for the sake of completeness. These internal derangements are outside the First Aider's diagnostic scope but you should be aware of them. The knee is the prize example. The knee joint contains four structures, which are as follows:

a. *The medial meniscus and (b) the lateral meniscus.* These menisci are commonly known as cartilages. The medial one lies on the medial side of the joint, (nearer the midline of the body). The lateral one lies on the lateral side of the joint, away from the midline of the body. They are both roughly 'new moon' shaped and their function is to facilitate rotational movements of the knee joint.

c. *The anterior cruciate ligament.* The function of this ligament is to prevent the femur from sliding too far backwards on the upper surface of the tibia.

d. *The posterior cruciate ligament* prevents the femur from sliding too far forwards on the upper surface of the tibia. These cruciate ligaments are so called because they cross over each other, within the joint. (Actually, from a strictly anatomical point of view, they are outside the knee joint proper, but that need not worry the First Aider. These ligaments *function* as an integral part of the knee joint). If any undue strain is placed upon the knee, then any of the four structures I have just mentioned can be damaged, whether there is any bony damage or not.

The medial and lateral collateral ligaments lie outside the knee joint, but they add stability and prevent the knee from bending in the wrong direction (see *Examination of the Knee*, in Part II).

The medial collateral ligament lies outside the medial (inner) aspect of the knee joint. It prevents the medial side of the joint from opening up, when a strain is applied to the fully-extended knee from the lateral (outer) aspect — i.e. it prevents the knee from bending so that the leg angles laterally (outwards). If the leg can be made to angle this way, then the medial collateral ligament has been torn.

The lateral collateral ligament functions similarly, by preserving the stability of the lateral side of the knee joint.

5. *Dislocation* is defined as 'complete loss of apposition of the articular surfaces of a joint' (i.e. complete loss of the normal relationship of one joint surface to another). You may have heard of the word '*Subluxation*'. This is a partial dislocation (i.e. incomplete loss of the normal relationship of joint surfaces).

Dislocation of the shoulder is quite common. It can be recognised by the following signs:

a. Flattened deltoid muscle (one of the 'give-away' signs described in Part II.)

b. Inability to touch the tip of the uninjured shoulder with the fingers of the hand of the same side as the injured shoulder (e.g. if the right shoulder is dislocated, the patient cannot touch the tip of his left shoulder with his right fingers).

Dislocation of the elbow is fairly common, and is easy to diagnose if you know the bony landmarks around the elbow. In this condition, the upper end of the ulna is pushed backwards with respect to the lower end of the humerus, and (unless the radius is fractured) the upper end of the radius is pushed upwards, with respect to the lower end of the humerus. The overall effect of dislocation of the elbow is shortening of the forearm. Shortening of the forearm can also be caused by fractures of the radius and ulna. Therefore, if you find a dislocation of the head of the radius (upper end) *without* dislocation of the upper end of the ulna (the olecranon process), you *must* search for a fracture of the shaft of the ulna, which would allow shortening of the forearm and, hence, dislocation of the head of the radius. Having warned you of this pitfall, I must confess that I have seen a few dislocations of the head of the radius without fracture of the ulna. In those cases, the only rational explanation can be that there was a subluxation of the inferior radio-ulnar joint (i.e. a partial dislocation of the joint between the lower ends of the radius and ulna, just above the wrist joint).

The bony landmarks of the elbow. Let us now indulge in a little practical amusement by finding these landmarks. If you cannot remember the names of these landmarks, it does not matter. The important thing is that you should be able to find them. You should always examine the patient's left elbow with your right hand, and his right elbow with your left hand. This is easy to remember because you cannot possibly touch your right elbow with your right hand, nor can you touch your left elbow with your left hand. Therefore, you can practise on your own elbows correctly. Apart from examining for a full range of movements at the elbow joint, we want to be able to find three things, *viz:*

a. the normal bony triangle of the elbow. If this is lost, then there is a dislocation or a fracture-dislocation of the elbow.

b. the normal position of the head of the radius. This normally rotates smoothly, when the forearm is pronated and supinated. If the head of the radius is tender, or if there is crepitus on pronation and supination, suspect a fracture of the head of the radius. If it is out of its normal position then it is dislocated.

c. any effusion which may be present.

a. *To find the bony triangle in your own left elbow*, first place your left elbow at a right angle, with the palm facing upwards. Now, place the palm of your right hand under the back of your left forearm, with the fingers pointing towards the left elbow. Slide your right hand towards the left elbow and when you reach the elbow, do the following three things:

i. With your right *Index* finger, find the 'point' of the elbow. This is the tip of the olecranon process of the ulna. Keep your right index finger on this point.

ii. With your right *middle* finger, search about on the medial side of the elbow (the side nearer to the body) and at about one or one-and-a-half inches away from the tip of the olecranon, you will find another bony point. This is the medial epicondyle of the humerus. Keep your middle finger on it.

iii. With your right *thumb*, search on the lateral (outer) side of the elbow and you will find another bony point, again about one or one-and-a-half inches away from the tip of the olecranon. This is the lateral epicondyle of the humerus. Keep your thumb on it.

With your thumb, index and middle fingers covering their respective bony landmarks, you will see that they form a triangle, because *when the elbow is flexed to a right angle*, they all lie in the same plane. If the elbow is fully extended, the triangle disappears, and all the points come to lie in a straight line. Try it! This should serve to remind you that the elbow must be at a right angle, if you are to find the bony triangle.

If you are examining someone else's left elbow, then hold his left hand in yours, as if shaking hands. Your left hand can then be used to hold his elbow at a right angle and your right hand is free to examine the elbow.

b. *To find the head of your own left radius*, simply find the lateral epicondyle of the humerus (the one you found with your right thumb, before) and place the tip of your right middle finger onto it, with your right fingers pointing towards your left shoulder. If you now place the tip of your right index finger next to the tip of the middle finger, you should feel the head of the radius. When you rotate your left forearm (i.e. pronate and supinate it) you will feel the head of the radius rotate beneath the tip of your right index finger. When practising this on someone else, you should use your left hand to rotate his left forearm by the 'hand shaking' method, and your right hand to rotate his right forearm.

c. *Effusions*, when present, produce a bulging of the capsule of the elbow joint. This bulging can be felt either between the tip of the olecranon and the medial epicondyle, or between the tip of the olecranon and the lateral epicondyle, when the elbow is held at a right angle.

With a little practice you should be able to find the normal bony triangle, the head of the radius and any effusion present in about ten seconds flat, if not less. You have no excuse for not practising how to find the bony landmarks. You have two hands and two elbows, and where you go, they go!

Dislocation of the patella is not uncommon and is often *recurrent* (i.e. the patient will tell you that it has happened previously). The patella slips laterally (i.e. towards the outer side of the knee, away from the midline of the body). Quite often, it slips back into its normal position when the knee is straightened. If it does, all well and good – just apply a bandage for support. If it does not slip back into position spontaneously you must *not* try to force it back.

6. *Fracture-dislocation* is dislocation associated with a fracture, or fractures. Good examples of fracture-dislocation occur in the shoulder, elbow and hip. Sir Percival Pott, who was a surgeon in London in the eighteenth century, described a fracture-dislocation of the ankle joint. This came to be known as 'Pott's Fracture'. Unfortunately, the term 'Pott's Fracture' has been used far too loosely for far too long. Nowadays, people often use the term quite wrongly, to describe any type of fracture or fracture-subluxation of the ankle joint (i.e. a fracture of the ankle joint with incomplete dislocation). Therefore, the term 'Pott's Fracture' is best avoided unless you are absolutely sure that the ankle is

a. *fractured* and
b. *dislocated*.

Dislocation and fracture-dislocation of the hip can both be caused by the same kinds of accidents (car crashes, coal-mining and mountaineering accidents). In either case, the hip may be flexed, adducted and internally rotated (as described in Part II). X-ray films are needed to differentiate dislocation from fracture-dislocation of the hip. This is an important point. The mechanism of injury involved in the production of dislocation of the hip is quite different from the mechanism of injury by which a fracture-dislocation occurs. Because of these differences in mechanism of injury, the methods of manipulation of these two injuries are quite different. So, without X-ray films, we do not know which method of manipulation to use. In any case, the manipulation of a hip joint can be very difficult. THEREFORE, ON NO ACCOUNT MUST YOU EVER TRY TO MANIPULATE A HIP JOINT!

The signs of fracture-dislocation of the shoulder and the elbow are the same as for dislocation. The fractures are usually noticed on X-ray films. Fracture-subluxation of the ankle joint is fairly common, whilst fracture-dislocation (the true Pott's Fracture) is very rare indeed. Dislocations of the joints of the fingers and thumbs are fairly common, and the deformity is usually quite obvious. Dislocation of the knee joint (as opposed to dislocation of the patella) is very rare.

7. *Pulled elbow* is a condition which occurs in young children. It is a

very painful injury and, if not treated early, the child will remain in pain and be unable to use the affected limb for a few days. The injury is caused by a jerking force along the fully-extended upper limb, and this causes the radius to slide away from the humerus. As it slides away from the humerus, the head of the radius becomes wedged into the annular ligament. Now, this annular ligament is a circular, tough ligament. It is attached to the upper end of the ulna, and normally it encircles the neck of the radius (the part just below the head of the radius). Its *normal* function is to prevent the upper end of the radius from splaying away from the upper end of the ulna, whilst at the same time allowing the radius to rotate freely. In the case of a 'pulled elbow', the function of the annular ligament is abnormal, because the head of the radius is wedged firmly into it. Thereby, free rotation of the radius has been lost, and any attempt to rotate the radius causes severe pain.

The history is usually obtained from the parents. They may tell you that the child was holding a rail when he fell, still holding the rail. Very commonly, the mother will tell you that they were walking along the pavement, hand in hand, when the child slipped off the edge of the kerb, and she pulled him up by the hand to prevent him from falling into the road. In either case, the mechanism of injury is a jerking force acting along the fully-extended upper limb and the result is the same. The child lets the injured limb hang limply to his side and he will not even *attempt* to use it, no matter how you coax him. If you ask his mother to take a firm grip on his *un*injured arm and then offer him a chocolate or a toy, he will struggle to try to free his uninjured arm, rather than try to use the injured one. If he had a greenstick fracture of the clavicle, or upper end of humerus, or lower end of radius, he would *at least try* to use the injured limb. The child himself, is usually crying, or may cry intermittently, and he usually complains of pain at the elbow. Sometimes however, he complains of pain at the wrist. This is because the sliding movement of the radius has not only wedged the head of the radius into the annular ligament, but it has also caused a subluxation of the inferior radio-ulnar joint (i.e. the joint between the lower ends of the radius and ulna, just above the wrist joint).

The diagnosis of 'pulled elbow' is made from the history, which is typical, and from the finding of a limp, loosely-hanging upper limb, which the child refuses to use. The treatment is by manipulation, which must NEVER be performed before an X-ray has been taken to rule out the possibility of a fracture.

3. *Estimation of potential blood loss from fractures.*

In Part I, I stated that broken bones bleed. I pointed out that the blood which oozes out of a broken bone into the tissues is lost from the circulation, just as surely as if it had poured onto the ground. Loss of blood from the circulation affects the general condition of the patient and the greater the blood loss, the greater its effect on the general condition. As this blood loss takes place over a few hours, it may take a few hours for the patient's general condition to deteriorate, but deteriorate it will, especially in a patient with multiple fractures. Just how rapidly we can expect a patient's general condition to deteriorate after injury depends on an estimation of *the total potential blood loss*. This estimation helps us to determine our order of priority of evacuation, when dealing with mass casualties. The general condition of the patient with the greatest *potential* blood loss can be expected to deteriorate faster than the general condition of the other injured people, and this gives him priority of evacuation over them. The following list is a good guide to the estimation of the total blood loss of an injured person:

	Estimation of potential Blood Loss
Fracture of:	
Clavicle	$\frac{1}{4}$ pint
Humerus (any part)	$\frac{1}{2} - 1$ pint
Forearm bones (one or both)	$\frac{1}{2} - 1$ pint
Hand & Wrist	usually negligible
Spinal bones	usually negligible
Pelvis	$2 - 4$ pints
Grossly fractured, unstable pelvis	up to 8 pints
Femur (any part)	$2 - 3$ pints
Tibia (any part)	$1 - 2$ pints
Fibula	$\frac{1}{4}$ pint
Foot (any part)	$\frac{1}{4}$ pint
Ankle	$\frac{1}{4} - \frac{1}{2}$ pint

I must emphasise that the above list is a *guide*. You may have seen similar lists, and you may have noted one or two discrepancies between those lists and this one, but please remember that these are estimates and not exact measurements. In any case the discrepancies between this list and any other should not be very great. So, please do not argue about which list is right and which is wrong. There is no exact right and wrong in an estimate of any kind, since, by definition, an estimate is a reasonably accurate assessment of something.

In practice, I use this list in the following way. I list the fractures found, add up the *potential minimum* and the *potential maximum* blood loss from them, and then take a figure half-way between the two totals. This figure I accept as the total potential blood loss of that person. This figure is also the number of pints of blood I would request for transfusion into that person. For example, if the minimum estimate is six pints and the maximum is ten pints, the figure half-way between these two is eight pints. So, I would accept eight pints as his potential blood loss and I would request eight pints of blood for transfusion into him. His response to the blood transfusion will determine whether or not he needs any more blood after the first eight pints.

Before I leave the subject of blood loss estimation, I should point out that blood loss within the abdomen or chest may have to be taken into account, too. I would also remind you of Air Hunger (see *Facial Appearance* Part II) and of the fact that the spleen carries a reserve supply of red blood cells which can be released into the circulation in an emergency (see Part I).

People with multiple fractures should be monitored prior to evacuation to hospital. The pulse, blood pressure and respiration should be *recorded*, preferably every fifteen minutes, up to the time of evacuation of that person. I shall elaborate on this, when I deal with 'Mass Casualties'.

Relief of pain in fractures and dislocations is rather a moot point at present. Many First Aiders have asked me about this, either because they are worried about having to give an injection, or about what they would have to inject. There could also be legal problems in allowing a First Aider to carry any potential drug of addiction, such as morphine or pethidine. Quite frankly, my own view is that First Aiders do not need to give injections, nor do they need to carry around dangerous drugs. There is a drug on the market now, which is called pentazocine hydrochloride (trade name 'Fortral') and this drug can be obtained in the form of suppositories. These are easily inserted into the rectum, well absorbed from the rectum and there is no problem about sterility, as there is with injections. Furthermore, pentazocine hydrochloride is not classed as a dangerous drug, and it is as strong a pain-killer as morphine. The only drawback is that it has a morphine-like action on the pupils (it causes the pupils to constrict). Therefore it must *not* be given to anyone who has sustained a head injury. Pentazocine hydrochloride is available as suppositories, 50 mg each, and also as injections, 30 mg and 60 mg per ampoule.

In all fairness to those who prefer to use the more traditional pain-killers, I should make mention of morphine, pethidine and papaveretum (Trade name, 'Omnopon'). All three of these are derived from opium. Opium is not one chemical compound, but a mixture of chemical compounds. Morphine and pethidine are pure chemical compounds derived from opium. They are strong pain-killers, but have a tendency to cause vomiting. However, they do have a sedative effect, not possessed by pentazocine hydrochloride. Papaveretum is a mixture of compounds derived from opium. It is as good a pain-killer as morphine and pethidine, has a better sedative effect and does not cause vomiting to the same extent. Morphine, pethidine and papaveretum tend to depress blood pressure, whereas pentazocine hydrochloride tends to cause a slight increase in blood pressure. Morphine is available in ampoules of 10 mg, 20 mg and 30 mg; Pethidine in ampoules of 50 mg and 100 mg, and papaveretum in ampoules of 10 mg and 20 mg. Legally, only doctors and certain members of the nursing profession are allowed to be in possession of drugs derived from opium, apart from pharmacists who are allowed to stock these drugs, and certain specialised First Aiders.

I have mentioned but a few of the many pain-killing drugs available.

To specialised First Aiders, who are likely to have to administer such drugs, I would suggest that they contact a doctor in their own area for further information and advice.

CHEST INJURIES

I must begin this section with a brief description of the anatomy of the chest, so that confusion can be avoided as you read on. The chest is a bony cage, capable of expansion and contraction. This cage is formed by the ribs, which are attached to the thoracic (or dorsal) vertebrae at the back, and to the sternum (or breastbone) at the front. The ribs afford a certain amount of rigidity to the chest wall and protection for the lungs, whilst at the same time allowing mobility to the chest wall. The gaps between the ribs are filled with muscles, called intercostal muscles, each of which is attached to the rib above and the rib below. In the right side of the chest, there is the right lung and in the left side of the chest, there is the left lung. The lungs are separated from each other by a space which runs down the middle of the chest called the *mediastinum*. This space contains the heart and great arteries and veins, lymph vessels and lymph nodes, trachea (windpipe) oesophagus (gullet), the vagus nerves and sympathetic nerve plexuses. The vagus nerves are cranial nerves (they originate in the brain) and they supply all parts of the alimentary tract. The sympathetic nerve plexuses are part of our autonomic nervous system (the nervous system which functions without our conscious control) and they are found in both thorax and abdomen. Each lung is separated from the chest wall by two layers of *pleura*. One layer of pleura covers the outer surface of the lung and the other layer covers the inner surface of the chest wall. Between the two layers of pleura, there is a thin film of lubricating fluid, so that the two layers of pleura can slide smoothly over each other as the chest expands and contracts.

Landmarks of the chest

At the top of the sternum there is a notch and, quite naturally, it is called the *sternal notch*. This notch lies between the left and right sterno-clavicular joints – the joints formed between the inner ends of the clavicles and the sternum. Find your own sternal notch and place the tip of your index finger on top of it. Now, push your finger backwards over the sternal notch, and the tip of your finger will hit your trachea. Normally the trachea is placed centrally behind the sternal notch. Any deviation of the trachea to left or right indicates that something is wrong. Now, run your index finger downwards until you are about one to one-and-a-half inches below the sternal notch. Here, you will feel a ridge running horizontally across the sternum. This ridge is called the *sternal angle*. If you follow the ridge to the left, you will find that it is exactly in line with a rib. This is the *second left rib*. Likewise on the right you will find that the sternal angle is exactly in line with the *second right rib*. By counting downwards from the second rib, on either side you can find the sixth, seventh, eighth, tenth rib etc. If you find a tender rib you can also count upwards from that rib until you reach the second rib, add one to the number you have counted, and that is the number of the injured rib.

One more landmark remains to be found in the chest, and this is the *apex beat*. The apex beat is the position on the chest wall at which the greatest impulse can be felt when the heart contracts. This position is normally in the fifth left intercostal space in the midclavicular line. The *intercostal spaces* are the gaps between the ribs. The fifth intercostal space is below the fifth rib. Find this space for yourself by counting downwards from the second rib. The *midclavicular line* is an imaginary line which passes downwards perpendicularly from the midpoint of the clavicle. It usually passes through the nipple, and for this reason, it is often called the 'nipple line'. However, where the left midclavicular line crosses the fifth left intercostal space, you should find your own apex beat. In very slim, lanky people, the apex beat is often found in the sixth left intercostal space in the midclavicular line. In people who have congenital heart abnormalities, the apex beat may be found in an unusual place. In the condition called *situs inversus*, the apex beat is on the right side of the chest. Fortunately, *situs inversus* is rare and people with it are usually quite healthy. Now that you know your way around the normal chest, we can proceed further.

Injuries to the chest

Apart from the fact that chest injuries can be painful, their importance is that they can be detrimental to the general condition of the patient because of

a. impaired lung function;
b. impaired heart function and
c. blood loss within the chest.

The types of chest injury can be broadly divided into *penetrating* wounds (where a sharp object pierces the chest wall) *blunt* injury (from a blow or fall) and *crushing* injury (if a man is trapped between a wall and a lorry).

A penetrating wound usually causes the lung on the side of the injury to deflate. If the wound is large enough, and it need not be very large, then air will pass through the wound into the chest when the injured person tries to breathe in, and out again when he tries to breathe out. Unfortunately, this can cause the mediastinum to move to-and-fro, from side to side. This movement is known as *mediastinal flap*. It interferes with the function of the heart, causing *cardiogenic shock*, in which the patient is pale and sweating; his blood pressure is low and his pulse is weak and rapid, just as if he had suffered a coronary thrombosis. In fact, it is the same kind of shock as that which occurs in coronary thrombosis. If the patient had some kind of lung disease prior to the collapse of his lung through injury, he would almost certainly show *cyanosis* (blueness of the lips and fingernails), indicating impairment of lung function. Penetrating wounds of the chest can cause bleeding into the chest, but this is not usually very gross. Fortunately, penetrating wounds of the chest are relatively uncommon in peacetime, though they are common in wartime.

Blunt injuries of the chest are by far the commonest seen in peacetime. Someone trips and falls onto his chest, or is thrown onto a steering wheel in a car crash. Crushing injuries are not as common, but they can be as serious, if not more serious, than blunt injuries. The damage sustained from either of these two kinds of injury depends upon the amount of violence involved. The damage ranges from bruised ribs or sternum right through the range of fractured ribs, fractured sternum, bruised heart muscle, bruised lungs and gross bleeding inside the chest, to stove-in-chest. In the stove-in-chest injury, a segment of the chest wall moves inwards as the patient breathes in, and outwards as he breathes out (i.e. in the opposite direction to that in which it should move each time). This causes mediastinal flap and a great deal of respiratory distress to the patient. A severe blow to the chest (e.g. from a steering wheel in a car crash) can cause *surgical emphysema*. This is a puffy swelling above and behind the clavicles, and when you feel at it, as if playing the piano, it gives the sensation of a soft, crinkly, tissue-paper-like feeling. It is the soft-tissue crepitus to which I referred when I discussed bony crepitus in *Injuries to Bones and Joints*. This may not appear for twelve or twenty-four hours after the injury, but if found, it indicates a severe compression injury of the chest. Bleeding inside the chest (between the lungs and the chest wall) after a compression injury may be up to eight pints or more, and blood loss can occur inside the chest whether ribs are fractured or not.

One other injury which I will mention is *ruptured thoracic aorta*. This occurs as the result of a sudden, violent, twisting movement of the trunk. It is usually caused by being thrown from a motor cycle, although it can be caused by a mountaineering accident. The rupture of the aorta may extend down into the abdominal part of the aorta. The condition is usually fatal, unless the patient can be taken to a hospital with a special chest surgical unit. The diagnosis of ruptured thoracic aorta should be suspected:

a. When the history suggests a sudden, violent, twisting movement of the trunk, and

b. When the patient is shocked, in the absence of any other definite signs, or in the presence of relatively minor injuries.

It should also be remembered that an injury to the *lower* ribs may cause damage to organs inside the abdomen. This will be referred to in 'Abdominal Injuries'.

Finally, before we proceed to the examination of the chest, I will remind you that muscle-spasm occurs as a protective mechanism after injury. Just as muscle-spasm after a fracture of the femur can cause a shortening of the femur, so muscle-spasm can reduce the movement of part of the chest wall after injury. The whole object of muscle-spasm after injury is to reduce movement of the injured part to a minimum. This, in turn reduces pain to a minimum. In fact, muscle-spasm is our own built-in, self-splinting mechanism.

Examination of the chest

This is always preceded by the history of course, and we want to know:

    a. How the injury occurred;

    b. If the patient is conscious, ask:

       i. 'Where does it hurt you?' and

      ii. 'Does it hurt when you take a deep breath?'

    c. 'Has there been any previous chest trouble?'

Question b(ii) is designed to reveal whether or not a *sharp, stabbing pain* occurs when the patient breathes in, because this is typically the pain which occurs when a rib has been fractured.

Question (c) is a useful one to ask, because if, for example, a man has had one lung removed, then he will tell you right away and this can prevent you from looking foolish later on.

The examination of the chest is where our time-honoured quartet of Inspection, Palpation, Percussion and Auscultation really come into their own.

a. *Inspection*. First of all, look at the patient's face, whilst feeling at his pulse. This saves time. You can learn very quickly to note the facial appearance, rate and type of respiration, and rate, rhythm and volume of the pulse all in a very short space of time. Make a note of these three things. Next, look at the patient's chest either from directly in front of him or directly behind him, and note whether the chest moves equally when he breathes in and out. If one side of the chest moves *less* than the other, then that side is probably being restricted by muscle-spasm, which indicates a probable injury on that side. Under the heading of Inspection, we can also look for cyanosis.

b. *Palpation*. First of all feel for the trachea and apex beat. If these are displaced to one side, this may be due to a collapsed lung, or severe bleeding into the chest, or both. We have already 'sprung' the ribs in our initial head-to-toe examination, and we have made a note of any pain so produced. Find any tender rib or ribs, and count up from it or them, as I have already described. Press on the sternum from top to bottom to find if there is any tenderness there. Feel the neck, above and behind the clavicles for surgical emphysema. Make a note of any positive findings, e.g. 'Tender sternum and 5th and 6th left ribs. Surgical emphysema'.

c. *Percussion*. This is where we drum on the patient's chest.

To practise percussion, place your left middle finger on a table, so that the front of the end *joint* of the finger is pressed firmly against the table. Now, hold your right middle finger in a curved position as if it were a hammer. Then 'drum' or 'hammer' with the tip of your right middle finger on the back of the end joint of the left middle finger, letting the movement flow from the right wrist. By percussing in this way over the middle of the table, you should produce a hollow sound. If you percuss the table-top above one of the legs, you should produce a more solid sound. Percussing a wall, or a stone fireplace should produce an even more solid sound. Having practised percussion on the table, you can now practise it on the front of your chest, and, assuming that you have no gross lung disorder, you should produce a rather hollow note. This is the normal percussion note, and we refer to it as *Resonance*. It varies slightly from one individual to another, depending on the size and shape of the individual chest. When you practise percussion on another person's chest, you should *always* compare one part of the chest with the similar part of the other side – compare upper right front with upper left front and so on.

Hyper-resonance is a much more hollow sound than the normal resonance, and it indicates a collapse of a lung, or part of a lung.

Stony dullness is like the note obtained when percussing a stone wall. It indicates fluid in the chest, which, after injury is usually blood. A collection of blood within the chest is called a *Haemothorax*.

d. *Auscultation*. As I pointed out in Part II, you can hear normal breath sounds, either by placing the ear onto someone else's chest, or by the use of a stethoscope. The breath sounds are heard much more clearly if you ask the patient to breath in and out *through the mouth*. Again, compare upper right front with upper left front, lower right back with lower left back etc. You should listen, also, directly over any tender ribs, because if you hear crepitus (a loud crunching sound), this will confirm your suspicion of a fractured rib.

Let us summarise these steps in the examination of the chest by considering an example. Let us assume that we have found a man who has had a heavy fall onto the left side of the chest. On examination we might well find the following:

1. *Inspection* (General condition and appearance). Face pale; slight cyanosis of lips; cold, clammy skin; rapid thready pulse. These signs indicate

    a. impairment of lung function (because of the cyanosis) and
    b. shock (because of the other signs).

Inspection of the chest reveals that the left side of the chest barely moves, indicating that the injury is on the left side.

2. *Palpation*. We find that the left 5th and 6th ribs are tender. We may even feel crepitus as we press on the ribs. Also we find that the trachea and the apex beat are displaced a little to the right.

3. *Percussion*. We find that the percussion note is normal all over the right side of the chest. Over the upper part of the left side of the chest, there is hyper-resonance, and over the lower part of the left side of the chest, there is stony dullness.

4. *Auscultation*. We find that the breath sounds over the right lung are

normal, but the left side of the chest is devoid of breath sounds. We hear crepitus over the 5th and 6th left ribs.

From these findings we conclude that the diagnosis is:

1. Fractured 5th and 6th ribs, left side.
2. Collapsed left lung.
3. Haemothorax, left side (collection of blood).
4. Shock, because of the injuries and the blood loss.

I will leave this example for you to re-ponder, and I will offer you the following two reminders:

a. Hyper-resonance with diminished or absent breath sounds indicates collapsed lung.

b. Stony dullness with diminished or absent breath sounds indicates haemothorax.

Emergency tracheotomy. This is literally a life-saving operation, and it should not be undertaken lightly. Emergency tracheotomy is indicated when the airway is blocked, cannot be unblocked and there is cyanosis. It follows therefore, *that you must make every effort to clear the airway, before embarking on emergency tracheotomy.* Having tried to clear the airway, and having found it impossible to do so, you are left with no alternative but to perform emergency tracheotomy. For this you will need the following:

1. A *sharp* knife.
2. Sharp-pointed scissors.
3. An incompressible tube (preferably curved metal with a guard on one end).
4. The ability to count up to four.
5. COURAGE IN ABUNDANCE!

At a pinch you could manage without the scissors, and instead of a metal tube, you could use (say) the empty barrel of a ball-point pen. *Method.* The head and neck must be *fully* extended. To ensure this, place something behind the shoulders to act as a cushion with the patient lying flat. Place a finger on the 'Adam's apple' and slide your finger down the trachea. You will feel rings of cartilage in the trachea, below the 'Adam's apple'. Count your way down these rings until you find the gap between the third and fourth rings. Directly over this space make an incision across the front of the trachea. This incision *must* go through the full thickness of the skin. Having drawn blood, by cutting the skin, this is where you need the 'courage in abundance' to carry on! Either with the knife, or preferably with the *closed* pointed scissors stab between the third and fourth cartilaginous rings. If you have used the scissors, they can be opened to widen the incision through the wall of the trachea, and then can be twisted through a right angle and used in the same way to push the third and fourth rings of cartilage apart and allow the tube to be passed into the trachea. Once the tube has been inserted into the trachea, the scissors can be removed, and the patient should be able to breathe through the tube. The tube should be held in position by the best means available, and the following precautions should be taken:

a. Take care that the patient does not cough out the tube.

b. Take care that no foreign matter (e.g. blood) gets into the tube. A dampened swab over the end of the tube serves as a good filter for this purpose.

c. If possible suck out the tube regularly (if you have a suction apparatus).

I hope that you will never have to perform emergency tracheotomy. However, if you are ever faced with a situation which *demands* tracheotomy, then I hope you will have the courage to do what is necessary to save a life. Otherwise, the patient will surely die.

Some specialised first aiders are now being taught the technique of endotracheal intubation. This technique involves the passing of a lubricated rubber tube into the trachea via the mouth or nose. The part of the tube which enters the trachea, is surrounded by an inflatable cuff. When the tube is in position, the cuff is inflated. The inflated cuff bulges against the wall of the trachea and, therefore it keeps the tube in place, as well as preventing secretions from the nose and mouth from passing into the lungs. Thus, the cuff prevents the unconscious person from drowning in his own secretions, whilst the tube provides a secure airway.

Whilst endotracheal intubation can be very useful for dealing with a deeply unconscious person, it is by no means easy and special training is necessary in order to acquire the skill. Also, it *cannot* be used when the airway is blocked and cannot be unblocked. The *only* solution to that problem, as stated previously, is emergency tracheotomy. This must be performed by the person on the spot. When a person whose airway is blocked and cannot be unblocked begins to show cyanosis (i.e. go blue in the face), then that person has only about ten minutes to live. The only way to save the person's life is to bypass the blockage, by performing an emergency tracheotomy *immediately*, because it may take much longer than ten minutes to summon a doctor to the scene.

ABDOMINAL INJURIES

Penetrating injuries of the abdomen are uncommon in peacetime, but are common in wartime, and they may cause injury to any organ inside the abdomen. *Closed injuries* of the abdomen are far more likely to occur in peacetime. The organs most commonly damaged are the liver, spleen, kidneys, bladder and urethra (the tube through which urine flows from the bladder to the outside world). These organs are the ones most commonly injured, because they are relatively immobile within the abdomen. The stomach and intestines usually escape injury from a blow to the abdomen, because they are relatively mobile within the abdomen. It has been said that the rectum may be torn in association with a nasty pelvic fracture, but quite frankly it is a very rare occurrence.

The liver, spleen and kidneys are tucked away neatly in the upper part of the abdomen. They lie below the diaphragm, which separates the chest from the abdomen, and they are hidden by the lower ribs, with the exception of about the lower two thirds of each kidney. *The kidneys* lie in the loins at the back of the upper abdomen, and they cannot normally be felt. *The spleen* is about one-and-a-half times the size of a fist, and normally it cannot be felt as it is hidden by the left lower ribs. Similarly, the bulk of the *liver* is protected by the right lower ribs, and so the liver cannot normally be felt. However, by pressing under the right rib margin at the front of the abdomen, you may elicit tenderness which in turn would make you suspect a rupture of the liver. Similarly, pressure under the left rib margin at the front of the abdomen could elicit tenderness, which would raise your suspicion of a ruptured spleen. If, by pressing in the left loin, you were to find tenderness, you would suspect a ruptured left kidney. If you found tenderness in the right loin, you would suspect a ruptured right kidney. *The urethra* is attached fairly firmly to the lower surface of the pubic bone, which you can feel at the middle of the front of the lower end of the abdomen and which is part of the pelvis. For this reason, the urethra is more often injured than the *bladder* which lies in the 'pit' of the stomach, behind the pubic bone. The bladder is relatively fixed within the abdomen by virtue of the fact that it is necessarily attached to the urethra, which is attached to the pubic bone. A full bladder is more likely to be injured than an empty one, because the wall of the bladder is held in a more rigid state when the bladder is full, than when it is empty. You will not be able to feel an empty bladder, though you may be able to feel a full one. Tenderness in the abdomen, just above the pubic bone, indicates the probability of a ruptured bladder. Blood in the urine usually comes from a ruptured urethra though it may also come from a ruptured bladder.

As in other parts of the body, muscle-spasm occurs in the abdomen as a built-in splinting mechanism after injury. *Rigidity* is the term we use to describe muscle-spasm of the abdominal wall. Rigidity occurs because bleeding inside the abdomen irritates the peritoneum, which is the sensitive inner lining of the abdomen. After a fall onto the back, bleeding can occur from the muscles which cover the front of the lower thoracic and lumbar vertebrae and a collection of blood forms in front of those muscles and behind the peritoneum which covers the back of the abdomen. Such a collection of blood is called a *retroperitoneal haematoma* (retro – behind; peritoneal – referring to the peritoneum; haematoma – a collection of blood in an abnormal situation). A retroperitoneal haematoma can account for two to four pints of blood-loss. Therefore, it should be borne in mind as a possible diagnosis if you are confronted with a man who has fallen onto his back, is in shock and has generalised rigidity of the abdomen, in the absence of any other definite signs or obviously serious injury (compare this with ruptured thoracic aorta described in *Chest injuries*).

The following points are useful to remember when dealing with someone who may have a closed abdominal injury:

1. Visible bruising on the abdominal wall almost always indicates internal injury.

2. A fall onto the left lower ribs may damage the spleen or the left kidney.

3. A fall onto the right lower ribs may damage the liver or the right kidney.

4. A fall onto the back may damage the right or left kidney, or it may cause a retroperitoneal haematoma.

5. An injury to the pelvis may damage the urethra or bladder.

6. Absent bowel sounds, in the presence of abdominal tenderness and rigidity (especially if the patient is shocked) indicate internal injury. Absent bowel sounds, *without* abdominal tenderness etc. can occur after severe blood-loss, or immediately after being concussed.

7. Blood loss from internal abdominal injuries can be *catastrophic*. Hence the importance of suspecting and detecting abdominal injuries before it is too late and the patient dies pouring out blood internally. It is also important to satisfy yourself that a person has NOT sustained an abdominal injury, because that is one injury less to worry about.

8. A person with a damaged spleen may be standing or walking about when you first see him. Do not let the 'walking casualty' fool you into neglecting to examine his abdomen. To do so could result in his death!

I shall never forget the day when I was shown an X-ray film of the left ribs of an eighteen-year-old boy. I could see no fractures on the X-ray film, so I went to the boy and asked him what had happened. He said that he was a railway worker and that he had been walking along a railway track and had slipped. As he fell, his left lower ribs had landed heavily on one of the railway lines. His face was rather pale and on examination I found rigidity down the left side of the abdomen, tenderness under the left rib margin and absent bowel sounds. I had no hesitation in diagnosing a ruptured spleen, even though he had walked into the accident department. His spleen was removed forthwith, and I trust that he will live to a ripe old age.

History

When asking the patient how the injury happened, you should be trying to create a mental picture of the accident — the way in which he fell and how he landed (remember: 'The words, 'I fell' should ring a bell'). You should also ask him to show you where he feels pain and you should ask him whether or not he has had any abdominal operations. Make a note of his answers.

Examination of the abdomen

Once again our time-honoured quartet goes into action:

a. *Inspection.* (1) Assess his general condition by looking at his face, feeling the pulse and taking the blood pressure. It is important to record the blood pressure if at all possible. (2) Look for visible signs of bruising on the abdominal wall. (3) See whether the abdomen moves with respiration, which is normal, or if it is held rigidly, which is abnormal.

b. *Palpation.* (1) Make sure that your hands are warm, as cold hands will cause the abdominal muscles to tighten up. (2) Slide your hand *gently* around the abdomen. Only in this way will you be able to feel *rigidity* if it is present in any part of the abdominal wall. (3) Ask the patient to breathe deeply and slowly through the mouth. As he breathes out his abdomen will be as relaxed as it possibly can be. (4) Press gently but firmly all over the abdomen to elicit tenderness. Also try to push your finger ends under each rib margin. Do not forget to press in the loins below the ribs at the back to elicit kidney tenderness. (5) If you find tenderness, tell the patient to tighten his abdominal muscles and then press again. *If it hurts more* when you press on his tensed abdomen, then the tenderness is caused by bruising of the muscles of the abdominal wall. *If it hurts less* then the tenderness is inside the abdomen itself. (6) Tell him to breathe deeply again, and then test all over the front of the abdomen for *rebound tenderness.* To do this, press down firmly and slowly, then suddenly release your pressure. If this causes pain and a sudden contraction of the abdominal muscles which makes the patient wince, then that is rebound tenderness. It is caused by irritation of the peritoneum by bleeding. Bleeding inside the abdomen can track downwards, and so it is quite common to find tenderness under the rib margin and rigidity and rebound tenderness lower down the abdomen, but on the same side.

c. *Percussion.* In examining the abdomen, the First Aider can percuss over the lower part of the abdomen. If the bladder is full, then the area of the lower abdomen which covers the bladder will give a dull note, compared with the rest of the abdomen, which will give a drum-like, or 'tympanitic' note. If the bladder is empty, the whole of the abdomen should give a tympanitic note. Apart from this, percussion of the abdomen is not a great deal of help to the First Aider, and further discussion of it would only serve to confuse him.

d. *Auscultation.* At the start of the Part I, I told you to listen to bowel sounds by placing your ear against someone else's abdomen. So you should be able to recognise normal bowel sounds by now! When bleeding occurs inside the abdomen, it irritates the intestines. This causes the irritated segment of bowel to try to empty itself and so, at first you may hear *hurried* bowel sounds (i.e. bowel sounds occurring in quicker succession than normally). You may hear the odd *gurgling* sound at this stage too. Later when the bowel segment has almost emptied itself, slow, *tinkling* bowel sounds can be heard. Finally, when the bowel segment is empty, it ceases all movement and at this stage, no bowel sounds can be heard. The bowel sounds are said to be *absent.*

Let us now imagine that we are examining a man who has fallen onto his back. We find that his face is pale, his skin dry, his pulse bounding and his blood pressure is $\frac{160}{90}$ (i.e. he is displaying the 'adrenaline response', at this stage). We see that his abdomen is held rather rigidly and, on palpation we find tenderness in the right loin, and rigidity and rebound tenderness down the right side of the abdomen. After percussing the lower abdomen, we decide that the bladder is empty and on auscultation, we find that the bowel sounds are absent. The diagnosis which *must* be suspected here is that of *ruptured right kidney*, and that diagnosis stands until the abdominal surgeons prove otherwise. The patient should be taken to hospital as soon as possible, because once his adrenaline response passes off, his blood pressure could collapse dramatically, with dire consequences for the patient.

Please practise examination of the abdomen. It is important
a. to exclude abdominal injury, if there is none present, and
b. to find an abdominal injury, if one exists.

You cannot hope to find abdominal injuries unless you look, feel and listen to the abdomen.

PREGNANCY

Most books on First Aid describe 'Emergency Childbirth', but I have not yet found one which tries to improve the First Aider's knowledge of pregnancy. As a result of this, when confronted with a pregnant woman who has injured a limb, the First Aider tends, at best to feel lost and at worst, to feel panic, often when there is no need for either. The object of this Subject is to give the First Aider confidence through knowledge and to enable him to reassure the pregnant woman with a limb injury that her pregnancy is still intact. After all, it should be remembered that the human race has been reproducing itself for about half a million years, and pregnancy and labour are normal parts of the process of reproduction. It is true that doctors and midwives see pregnant women regularly at antenatal clinics, but in the majority of cases, their function is to reassure themselves and the mother-to-be that everything is proceeding *normally*. Similarly, during labour, the function of the doctors and midwives is to supervise labour in order to see that it is proceeding *normally*, and to intervene *only* in the few cases which do not go according to plan. Therefore, the first thing for the First Aider to learn is that pregnancy and labour are normal events in the calendar of human life, and that, in the vast majority of cases – Nature knows best!

General information about pregnancy
The average duration of pregnancy is forty weeks which is ten *lunar* months or two hundred and eighty days or approximately nine calendar months and one week. A useful point to remember is that three calendar months (e.g. from 15th June to 15th September) are thirteen weeks, roughly. Therefore nine calendar months are equal to thirty-nine weeks. The date on which the baby is due to be born is called the expected date of confinement (EDC) or the expected date of delivery (EDD). This is calculated as being forty weeks after the *first* day of the last *normal* menstrual period. I stress the word 'normal' because it is quite common

for a 'period' to occur after conception has taken place, but this period is not a normal one because it is usually of shorter duration than a normal period and it usually occurs later than a normal period would be expected to occur. In actual practice we calculate the EDC by taking the date on which the last normal period began, adding seven days and then adding nine calendar months (or subtracting three calendar months, which gives the same answer). For example:

	Example 1.	Example 2.
First day of last period	1st September	30th September
Add seven days	8th September	7th October
Add nine months	8th June	7th July
EDC	8th June	7th July

When the pregnant woman reaches her EDC she is said to be *at term*. After conception, the fertilised ovum is implanted into the inner lining of the womb, and at the site of implantation the 'afterbirth' or *placenta* develops. The placenta is essential for the survival of the unborn baby, because the baby is being incubated inside a sac of fluid within the mother's womb and therefore it cannot breathe in the normal way, nor can it forage for food. The baby is isolated in the fluid (liquor) contained in the bag of *membranes*. The baby's blood flows along the umbilical cord from the baby to the placenta, and then back to the baby. Likewise, the mother's blood flows through cavities in the wall of the womb next to the placenta. In this way oxygen and foodstuffs can pass from the mother's blood to the baby's blood through the placenta, and carbon dioxide and other excretory products pass from the baby's blood to the mother's blood. The placenta does not allow the mother's blood to mix with the baby's blood, because this could be disastrous for the baby, especially if its blood group were different from the mother's blood group. The baby is, then, entirely dependent upon the mother and the placenta for survival. If the placenta becomes detached completely from the wall of the womb, the baby will die by suffocation, because it will have lost its supply of oxygen.

The womb grows in size as pregnancy continues and at term, it is a large, powerful, muscular organ, ready to expel the baby during labour. During the last twelve weeks of pregnancy the mother feels the womb contract from time to time, but these are not painful contractions. They are known as Braxton-Hicks contractions, and they indicate that the womb is toning itself up in preparation for the hard work it will have to do during labour, when the force of its contraction reaches up to fifty pounds per square inch. I often wonder how babies survive such a force, but in fact they do. The womb provides protection for the growing baby, since any shock waves are dispersed through the liquor inside the womb. The womb also acts as an incubator for the baby and if a woman is in premature labour, the best baby-incubator in the world for transporting the baby to hospital is the womb itself.

As pregnancy advances, the baby grows steadily bigger. A woman who is having her first baby will feel *movements* any time from the twentieth week onwards (usually about the twenty-fourth week). These movements are caused by the baby's arms and legs as it moves itself about inside the womb. A woman who is having a second or third baby may feel these movements any time from the sixteenth week of pregnancy onwards. At twenty weeks the fundus (i.e. upper end of the womb) is up to the level of the navel, and the fundus can be found by pressing with the edge of the palm. If you begin near the top of the abdomen and then move your palm a little further down the abdomen before you press again, eventually by repeating this action, you will find the fundus. At the twenty-eighth week of pregnancy the fundus is about half way between the navel and the lower end of the sternum. At term it is up to the lower end of the sternum. If you are lucky enough to find a pregnant woman who will let you feel at her abdomen, then take the opportunity to do so (suitably chaperoned of course!), because such opportunities will not arise often for the First Aider. Similarly, if you have the chance to listen to an unborn baby's heart, then take it. The heart can usually be heard best by placing your ear to the mother's abdomen, either in the left lower or right lower part of the abdomen, depending on which way the baby is lying. The baby's heart can be heard faintly at twenty-eight weeks and as term is approached it becomes louder, and therefore much easier to hear. Its rate is about one hundred and twenty beats a minute.

If the baby is born before the thirty-fifth week of pregnancy its chances of survival are rather poor. From the thirty-fifth week up to the thirty-eighth week there is a sharp improvement in the survival rate. From the thirty-eighth week right through to the forty-second week the survival rate is the same − i.e. the baby has the same chance of survival whether it is born two weeks prematurely, two weeks overdue, or at term. If pregnancy continues beyond forty-two weeks the placenta begins to degenerate and the baby's chances of survival begin to fall quite sharply. Legally, an unborn baby is deemed to be capable of a separate, independent existence from the end of the twenty-eighth week of pregnancy onwards. We use this feature of the law to define abortion (commonly called 'miscarriage') and premature labour, as follows:

Abortion is defined as 'the expulsion of the products of conception (i.e. the baby and the placenta) *before* the end of the twenty-eighth week of pregnancy'. Abortion is the correct medical term for miscarriage. It should not be confused with *criminal* abortion, nor with legal termination of pregnancy.

Premature labour is defined as 'expulsion of the products of conception *after* the end of the twenty-eighth week of pregnancy and *before* term'.

The legal importance of these two definitions is that, when an abortion occurs there is no need to obtain a death certificate for the baby. However, when premature labour occurs and the baby dies, it is necessary by law, to obtain a death certificate for the baby, otherwise the person, or persons, concerned may be charged with *Concealment of birth* (under the law of England and Wales) or with either *Concealment of pregnancy* or *Child murder* (under Scottish Law). These are all serious offences.

Let us now consider Labour, Premature labour and Abortion, in that order.

Labour

In Britain, 80 per cent, or more, of babies are born in hospital, and the arrangements for hospital delivery are usually made well in advance of labour. There is no doubt in my mind that the safest place for any woman in labour is a proper maternity unit of a hospital. Therefore the first sensible thing to do for any woman at term and in labour is to warn the appropriate maternity unit (i.e. the one where she has been booked for confinement) by telephone so that the unit will prepare for her arrival. The second sensible thing to do is to get her to the unit as quickly and *safely* as possible. If the woman is booked for home confinement, she will be able to give you the telephone number of the midwife on call. If a woman is not booked for home or hospital confinement, then this means that she has not attended antenatal clinic as she should have done, and she is a very foolish woman indeed. Nevertheless, under these circumstances, the correct procedure is to contact the general practitioner on call, because he can arrange for her admission to hospital.

It would seem that I have left the First Aider very little to do, but it could happen that a First Aider arrives on the scene just as delivery of the baby is imminent and there is no time to take the mother to hospital. On a number of occasions it has happened that a baby has been born in an ambulance on the way to hospital, with an ambulanceman acting as midwife. So it will do you no harm to know what is going on during labour.

We can divide labour up into three stages. *The First Stage* of labour is that in which the neck of the womb is dilating, and the baby's head is being pushed steadily down into the pelvis. It may last for a few hours. *The Second Stage* is that in which the baby is pushed out (born) and it begins when the neck of the womb is *fully* dilated. This stage normally lasts for no more than one hour, although it may last for as little as ten minutes, especially if the woman has had babies previously. *The Third Stage* is that in which the placenta and membranes are delivered. Since it follows the birth of the baby, it explains why the placenta is often called the 'afterbirth'. This stage may be completed a few minutes after the second stage, or it may last up to an hour. You must *never* interfere with it or you may cause very severe bleeding. Having gained the basic information about labour, we can now consider each of the three stages of labour in rather more detail.

THE FIRST STAGE of labour begins with irregular, sharp, abdominal pains, sometimes accompanied by low backache. The mother passes a small amount of blood-stained mucus from the vagina and this blood-stained mucus is called a *Show*. The mucus has been released from the neck of the womb, where it has been acting as a barrier to keep out infectious germs during pregnancy. Every time the womb contracts, the mother feels a pain. If you place a hand on her abdomen you can actually feel the womb tighten up and relax, as the contraction builds up and as it passes off. The contractions (and the pains, too) gradually become stronger and last longer. The pattern of the contractions changes gradually from an irregular one to a regular one in which the contractions occur about every ten minutes. When this point is reached, the first stage of labour is said to be *established*. From this point onwards the contractions increase steadily in strength, frequency and duration.

As previously stated, these contractions serve to push the baby's head firmly into the pelvis and to dilate the neck of the womb. They also cause the membranes to bulge increasingly through the ever-widening neck of the womb, and eventually the membranes rupture, liberating a sudden gush of crystal – clear liquor. When this gush of liquor occurs you know that *the membranes have ruptured*. This may happen late on in the first stage or it may be delayed until the second stage of labour. When a woman is having her first baby it is quite common for the first stage to last twelve hours or more. Women who have had babies previously, tend to have shorter first stages and second stages too.

Actions in first stage

1. Encourage the woman to conserve her energy, because she will need it during the second stage. You can do this by:

    a. Telling her to relax between pains, by breathing slowly.

    b. Telling her to pant deeply and rapidly whenever she has a pain. This will help her to relax with pains.

    c. Telling her not to push in the first stage, because this will sap her strength and it could be positively harmful to her.

2. Fluid refreshment should be given but NOT solid food.

3. Every fifteen minutes record the time interval, in minutes, between the beginning of one contraction and the beginning of the next. For example, if this time interval is ten minutes, we would record it as 'contractions 1:10'. If it were six minutes we would record it as 'contractions 1:6.' This record not only provides us with a useful indication of the way in which the first stage is progressing, but it also shows the mother that she is not being neglected!

4. Record the time at which the Show is passed. If the Show was passed before you arrived on the scene, ask the mother when it was passed.

5. Record the time at which the membranes rupture.

THE SECOND STAGE of labour may last up to one hour, or it may be finished in ten minutes or less. It begins when the neck of the womb is *fully dilated* and this is indicated by:

1. very strong pains occurring every three minutes, and
2. an *irresistible* urge to push, felt by the mother, with each pain.

The mother is compelled to push with each pain, and gradually the baby's head becomes visible. When the widest part of the baby's head has reached the outlet of the vagina, the head is said to be *crowned*. Next, the rest of the head emerges, and having done so, the baby's head turns, so that it comes to face either directly to the mother's right side, or directly to the mother's left side, depending on the position of the baby's body, which is still inside the womb. It will be appreciated that, if the baby is facing to the mother's right side, the baby's right shoulder will lie towards the front of the mother and its left shoulder will lie towards the back of the mother. In this case, the right shoulder is said to be the *anterior shoulder*, i.e. the shoulder which is lying towards the anterior part (front part) of the mother. If the baby is facing towards the mother's left side, then the reverse is the case and the left shoulder is the anterior shoulder. It is important to ensure that the anterior shoulder is delivered before the other shoulder, otherwise the mother could sustain a rather bad vaginal tear. Once the anterior shoulder has emerged, the rest of the baby's body slips out quite easily. After the whole of the baby has been delivered, the umbilical cord continues to pulsate for about a minute or so. This pulsation can be felt by holding the cord *gently* between your thumb and fingers. When the cord stops pulsating, this marks the end of the second stage of labour.

Actions in second stage

1. When the mother feels a pain coming on, tell her to take a deep breath, hold it and push hard while the pain lasts.

2. Between pains, encourage the mother to relax as much as possible.

3. As the head of the baby crowns, tell the mother 'Don't push! Pant as hard as you can!' At the same time place your hand against the baby's head to guard against sudden expulsion of the head. If the baby's head is expelled suddenly, the mother may tear herself, and the baby could suffer brain damage.

4. The next move is to deliver the rest of the baby's head *between contractions* (between one pain and the next). So, when the head is crowned, and when the mother has panted until the pain has passed away, tell her to give a *gentle* push, whilst you are still exerting counter-pressure with your hand. This will allow the head to emerge gently, and the mother should sustain no more than a slight tear of the vagina. In fact, she will probably escape without a tear at all.

5. FEEL FOR THE CORD! This is very important. As soon as all of the baby's head has emerged, feel around the baby's neck for the cord, which may be wrapped around the baby's neck and which could strangle

the baby as the rest of the body is born. Therefore:

a. If the cord cannot be felt, you breathe freely and wait for the next pain.

b. If the cord is around the neck, hook a finger round it and pull until there is sufficient play in the cord to unwrap it from around the baby's neck.

c. If the cord is wrapped so tightly round the baby's neck that you cannot unwrap it, it must be ligated, divided and then unwrapped. To do this, select one part of the cord, slip two ligatures around it and tie them *tightly* about one inch from each other (shoe laces will do for ligatures). Next, cut the cord between the two ligatures, *taking care* not to cut any other part of the cord, or the baby's neck or face. The cord will now easily unwrap from the baby's neck. Should you have to ligate and divide the cord, it is important that the mother does not push until it has been done. Therefore, you must tell her to 'pant like mad' if she feels a pain, and not to push until you have ligated, divided and unwrapped the cord. You should complete this task with all possible speed, because the mother's patience and endurance of pain are both being stretched to the limit at this stage in the proceedings.

6. *With the next pain,* the anterior shoulder should be delivered. To do this, tell the mother to push and at the same time you should exert very *gentle* traction on the baby's head and neck. This traction should be exerted downwards and backwards in relation to the mother (i.e. downwards towards her feet and backwards towards her sacrum).

7. Once the anterior shoulder has emerged, cease the traction and allow the rest of the baby's body to slide out under the force of the mother's push. *The baby is now born. Make a note of the time of birth.*

8. Now, hold the baby upside down to allow any liquor and secretions to drain out of the mouth. The baby should begin to breathe and cry spontaneously. If necessary, smack it on the bottom to make it cry.

9. *When the cord stops pulsating* tie two ligatures *firmly* around the cord about one inch apart and a good six inches from the baby's navel area. Then divide the cord between the two ligatures. If you have had to divide the cord already (as in 5 c.) simply make sure that you tie a firm ligature six inches away from the baby.

10. Wrap the baby snuggly in a towel or a baby blanket, and then put the baby to the mother's breast. Putting the baby to the mother's breast does three things. First it pleases the mother and the sight of her baby gives her a sense of achievement at the end of her pregnancy. Secondly, it is comforting to the baby and gives it a feeling of security. Thirdly when the baby suckles on the mother's breast, it stimulates chemical activity within the mother, which tones up the womb for further contractions which cause expulsion of the placenta.

THE THIRD STAGE OF LABOUR commences when the cord has stopped pulsating, and it ends when the placenta and membranes have been expelled *completely*. This stage commonly lasts half-an-hour, although it may be as little as ten minutes, or up to an hour. After expulsion of the baby, the womb takes a well deserved rest, and it is important that you allow the womb to rest. In third stage the golden rule is NO UNNECESSARY INTERFERENCE. I cannot stress this too strongly because third stage interference is the greatest cause of third stage haemorrhage! So, be patient and let Nature take its course.

It will be appreciated that, once the womb has expelled the baby, it will contract down because it has emptied itself of a large proportion of its burden. The fundus of the womb should now be just below the level of the mother's navel, and it should feel firm. Having satisfied yourself of this, *keep your hands off the fundus!* You will also realise that the part of the cord which is still attached to the placenta, is visible at the vagina from which it is protruding. We now wait for the *three signs of separation of the placenta*, which are:

    a. the fundus rises

    b. the cord lengthens

    c. fresh bleeding occurs from the vagina

    a. The fundus of the womb rises and falls repeatedly, but the general trend is for the fundus to move upwards towards the navel. This causes bleeding to occur between the placenta and the wall of the womb, which separates the placenta from the wall of the womb.

    b. As the placenta is pushed downwards within the womb, so more of the cord emerges from the vagina, causing an increase in the length of the cord outside the vagina.

    c. The fresh bleeding comes from the bleeding which separates the placenta from the wall of the womb.

When these three signs occur, they indicate placental separation. As they occur, the mother feels another pain in her abdomen and the desire to push returns. As she pushes, she expels the placenta, membranes and blood, and after this the womb contracts down firmly and the bleeding stops. Labour is now finished. It is normal to lose up to one pint of blood during third stage, but more than one pint of blood-loss is abnormal. For this reason, it is important to have some form of receptacle in which the blood can be collected as it leaves the vagina so that the amount of blood lost can be measured. The placenta and membranes are usually collected in the same receptacle and it is important to preserve them, so that a doctor or midwife can inspect them later to ensure that they have expelled completely. If part of the placenta or membranes have been retained inside the womb, secondary haemorrhage may occur later on, or infection may supervene after a few days. So, preserve the placenta for inspection.

Actions in third stage

    1. Wait. NO UNNECESSARY INTERFERENCE! I re-emphasise this.

    2. Watch for the signs of placental separation.

    3. Have a receptacle ready to receive the placenta, membranes and blood.

4. After the mother has pushed out the placenta and membranes, *feel for the fundus*. The fundus should be about half way between the navel and the pubic bone and it should feel firm.

5. Preserve the placenta and membranes for inspection (preferably in a plastic bag).

6. Measure the amount of blood lost. If you cannot measure it then preserve it for measurement later on.

7. Make a note of the time the placenta and membranes were expelled.

8. Tell the mother to cross her legs. This restricts any oozing of blood from a vaginal tear, if she has sustained one.

9. Ensure that the mother is warm and comfortable (and baby too.)

10. Brew up! Mother has earned a nice cup of tea – and so have you! In any case, the mother should not be moved for at least an hour after the end of third stage, and one or two cups of tea help to replace the volume of blood lost during third stage, apart from making her feel refreshed.

I hope that you can now understand what goes on during a normal labour and I hope that you realise that there is nothing very terrible about being at a normal delivery. After all, it is the mother who does all the hard work! What she needs most of all from you is encouragement, confidence and reassurance. If you find the foregoing description of labour and its management too hard to remember, then just remember the following important points:

1. Give the mother encouragement and reassurance.

2. No pushing in First Stage. Mother must pant with pains.

3. Encourage mother to push with pains in Second Stage.

4. The baby's head must be delivered *between* contractions (i.e. between pains).

5. *Feel for the cord* as soon as the baby's head is delivered.

6. The baby's body must be delivered *with* a contraction and NEVER between contractions. If you deliver the body between contractions, you may cause serious, even fatal, bleeding from the womb.

7. Wait for the signs of placental separation. No interference in Third Stage.

8. Collect and preserve the placenta, membranes and blood.

9. Keep mother and baby warm and comfortable after delivery.

10. Brew up the tea. You must not forget that!

Premature labour

More often than not, premature labour occurs for no obvious reason. Occasionally, it occurs because of weakness of the neck of the womb. Sometimes spontaneous bleeding occurs between the placenta and the wall of the womb causing separation of part, or all, of the placenta from the wall of the womb. Such spontaneous bleeding is called *Accidental haemorrhage*, although it usually occurs spontaneously and *not* because of injury sustained by the mother. In fact, although I have seen many pregnant women who have fallen downstairs, or who have been involved in road accidents, I have seen only one woman who, by falling directly onto her abdomen, had caused separation of the placenta and hence the death of her baby. As I stated previously, the womb affords the baby great protection and although many pregnant women sustain injuries by falling, the vast majority of unborn babies come to no harm whatsoever.

On the stage, on television and in films, it quite often happens that 'our heroine' loses her baby as a result of falling downstairs. In real life this is a very rare occurrence indeed, even if the mother does fall downstairs.

Accidental haemorrhage, then, is spontaneous bleeding between the placenta and the wall of the womb. It causes muscle-spasm in the wall of the womb at the site of the bleeding and if you press on that part of the womb, you will find tenderness, though the rest of the womb will not be tender. As you might expect, accidental haemorrhage can trigger off premature labour.

The last cause of premature labour which I will mention is the death of the unborn baby (the technical term for this is *'fetal death in utero'* or FDIU for brevity). If for any reason the unborn baby dies in the womb, its death is soon followed by the onset of labour, presumably because there is no future in incubating a dead baby. The signs of FDIU are

1. the womb ceases to increase in size as it normally does during pregnancy.

2. the mother ceases to feel movements and

3. the baby's heartbeat can no longer be heard.

The symptoms, signs and stages of premature labour follow roughly the same pattern as those of labour at term, except that where premature labour has been brought on by accidental haemorrhage, the first symptom may be a severe pain localised to one part of the womb and the first signs may be vaginal bleeding (from the haemorrhage inside the womb) associated with localised tenderness and rigidity of one part of the womb. Usually, the baby is delivered before the placenta, but in premature labour sometimes the placenta may be delivered before the baby, in which case the baby will be stillborn. Blood loss in premature labour is not usually severe, but occasionally it can be.

Actions in premature labour

The mother must be taken to a hospital which has a Premature Baby Unit, where incubators are available for premature babies. No matter how far on in labour the mother appears to be, her womb is still the best incubator in which to take the baby to hospital. If you can contact her doctor first, do so, because he will arrange for her admission in the correct manner. However, if you are way out in the wilds of nowhere, just strap the mother to a stretcher and get moving! If the baby happens to be born on the way to hospital, wrap it up and keep it as warm as you can. Do not forget to ligate and divide the cord and preserve the placenta and membranes for inspection, if they are expelled.

Abortion ('Miscarriage')

About one pregnancy in five ends as an abortion and it is usually found to be due to the fact that there was some fault in the fertilised ovum, which would have resulted in some serious defect in the baby had the pregnancy continued to term. No blame can be attached to the parents for the fault in the fertilised ovum. It just happens that these faults occur from time to time because human reproduction is not one hundred percent perfect. We can regard spontaneous abortion as Nature's way of filtering out the defects during the early part of pregnancy, rather than allowing the human defects to be born at term with little or no chance of survival. It is true that some babies are born with defects of the heart, brain, limbs, nervous system etc., but the fact that the vast majority of human beings are born in perfect health shows just how well Nature's filtering system works.

Symptoms of abortion. These may commence in any order. They are:

a. *Vaginal bleeding.* This is often the first sign. It may be very slight at first and then become heavier. The mother often passes clots of blood and in all, abortion may result in the loss of a few pints of blood.

b. *A 'fleshy' substance* may be passed, often with the clots of blood. You should ask the mother if she has passed a fleshy substance. If she has, then it should be retained for inspection if it is still available, because this fleshy substance is probably the *ovum*.

c. *Low backache.* This is often quite severe and it may be the first symptom.

d. *Low abdominal pains.* If the woman has had a baby previously, she will tell you that these pains are like labour pains, and in fact they are caused by contractions of the womb. The pains become regular and they increase in strength and frequency, just like labour pains.

Signs of abortion (a) *The ovum* (the fleshy substance) may be available to see. (b) *Vaginal bleeding* can be seen. (c) *Tenderness of the womb* can be elicited by pressing just above the pubic bone.

Actions

The mother must be taken to hospital because blood-loss can be very heavy. Preferably, contact her doctor who will arrange for her admission, but again, if you are out in the wilds, just get going. The best possible thing that you can do for the woman is to get her to hospital. You will do her not one scrap of good by keeping her away from hospital and the baby is doomed to die, anyway.

By now you should have a reasonable understanding of pregnancy and you should be able to understand that, if you find a pregnant woman who has been injured, then provided that:

1. There is no vaginal bleeding.
2. There is no abdominal pain.
3. There is no low backache.
4. There is no tenderness of the womb when you press around the abdomen.

5. The woman can feel movements (if she is far enough on in pregnancy).

6. The baby's heartbeat can still be heard (depending on the stage of pregnancy);

then it follows that the pregnancy is still intact!

So there is no cause for alarm as far as the pregnancy is concerned. It is important to reassure the woman about this *forthwith*.

MASS CASUALTIES

It does not take much imagination to realise that disasters can occur anywhere and at any time. The Police have the ultimate responsibility for dealing with disasters and each Police force already has contingency plans for dealing with disasters in its own area. Even when only one person is lost or injured, the Police accept responsibility for the search for and the rescue of that person, even though the actual search and rescue may be carried out by a civilian Search and Rescue Team. It follows, therefore, that if a person is lost or injured, or if mass casualties have occurred, the Police *must* be informed without delay, because the Police are in the best position to contact rescue teams, ambulance chiefs, fire brigade chiefs and hospitals.

The search for survivors in out-of-the-way places and the evacuation of those survivors should be conducted under the guidance of the most experienced mountaineer, fell-walker, potholer, etc. He is usually the Team Leader, anyway. Once the scene of the accident is reached, the most experienced First Aider should be given a free hand, and he may not be the Team Leader. The most experienced First Aider is the one who is the best at diagnosis, and he should be given a title to denote this. Let us call him the Chief First Aider. The Chief First Aider should have a group of trusted First Aiders to whom he can delegate duties and he should be well aware of the individual capabilities of each one of his First Aiders. The first thing to do is to clear the accident site as much as possible by telling two or three of his First Aiders to usher the walking casualties to one side. These First Aiders will then have the duty of going over all of the walking casualties from head-to-toe, recording names, ages, addresses, religion, next-of-kin, and any injuries found, as well as making sure that each casualty has no internal injury before he is finally and confidently declared to be a walking casualty. The exclusion of internal injury in someone who was walking when found is an important job and if one of the First Aiders suspects an internal injury, he should report his suspicion to the Chief First Aider, who can then check the findings.

Whilst the walking casualties are being checked over systematically, the Chief First Aider and the rest of the First Aiders should go to work on the non-walking casualties. A useful time-saving measure would be for each First Aider to have with him another member of the team, *who can write legibly*, so that he can act as a clerk to the First Aider recording name, age, etc., and any injuries found, which would be dictated to him by the First Aider. By this method, a lot of people can be examined from head-to-toe and have their injuries recorded in a relatively short space of time. I stress again the importance of head-to-toe examination of every casualty *before* he is evacuated from the accident site. A suggested casualty record card is shown on the following page.

The Chief First Aider should soon be in possession of a list of injuries for each person. He can then check quickly for himself those who have the worst injuries and, having done so, the Chief First Aider must decide on his priority of evacuation. It is his duty, his decision and his responsibility alone. He is the one who is at the scene of the accident and who can see for himself the state of the injured people.

If there is only one stretcher available, he must decide on the one person who needs to be given priority of evacuation, and this may be very difficult indeed. The Chief First Aider must make that decision and make it quickly, otherwise the rescue operation will be held up. When the decision has been made then it stands, whether it is right or wrong. Let there be no dissension in the ranks! If there is dissent, the rescue operation will assume a negative attitude; but if the Chief First Aider's decisions are arrived at quickly and adhered to, then the stretcher parties can get on with their job and the attitude of the whole rescue team will remain positive.

If there are, (e.g.) three stretchers available immediately, then the burden on the Chief First Aider is eased somewhat, because he can decide which three people are the most badly injured without having to decide which of these three people is in the worst condition. He simply tells the Team Leader who those three people are, and the Team Leader puts his stretcher parties to work. I shall return to the Chief First Aider's duties later.

The Team Leader is in overall command of his team during the rescue operation. There is no doubt about that! If the Team Leader gives an order, then all other team members *must obey*, because the Team Leader is responsible for the safety of his team. The Team Leader is also responsible for the evacuation of casualties and this poses the problem of evacuating the walking and the non-walking casualties. Obviously, when the non-walking casualties are ready the stretcher parties will waste no time in getting to work, because *speed of evacuation is vital*! This means that casualties should be transported as quickly *and as comfortably* as possible. If a person with a chest injury or an abdominal injury is transported rapidly and roughly, his general condition can deteriorate very quickly. This applies particularly to the mountain rescue situation, where speed of evacuation, comfort and the casualty's general condition must all be carefully assessed, so that the casualty eventually arrives at hospital in the shortest possible time commensurate with the least possible deterioration in his general condition.

If the Team Leader waits until all the non-walking casualties have been

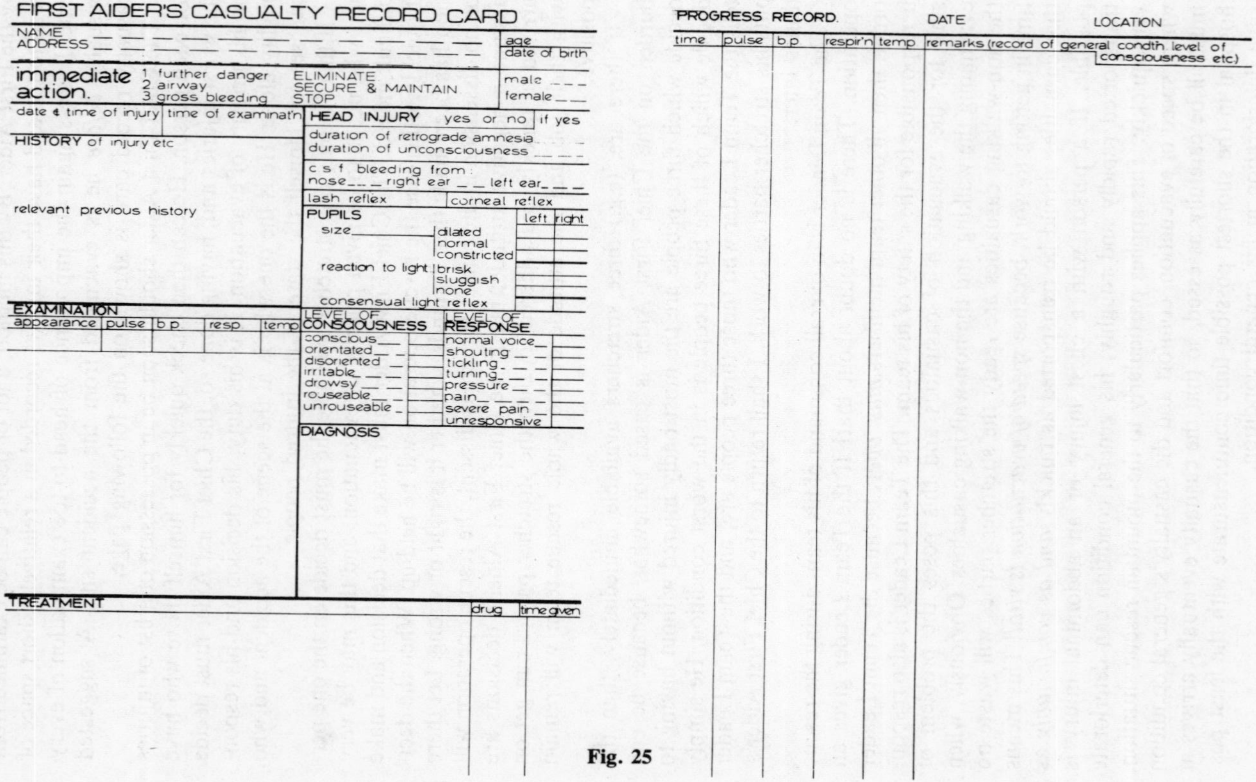

Fig. 25

evacuated before he starts to evacuate the walking casualties, he may find that by this time, some of the walking casualties have begun to suffer hypothermia and may need a stretcher after all. Not only is this bad for the casualties but it is rather fatiguing for the stretcher parties! Therefore, I would *suggest* that the Team Leader divides his team members into stretcher parties and escort groups.

When the first half dozen or so of the walking casualties have been checked over to ensure that they are fit to be evacuated on foot, then it would need only two team members to escort them to safety, one in the lead and one bringing up the rear. Two more members could escort the next half dozen walking casualties whilst the first two were returning to the accident site. Preferably, the Team Leader should choose one evacuation route for the stretchers and a different route for the walking casualties, but it does not really matter if they all use the same route, provided that the walking casualties do not impede the progress of the stretcher parties.

Having begun the evacuation of the casualties, let us now return to the duties of the Chief First Aider. He has already decided on (let us say) his first three priority casualties, because they are already being evacuated by the stretcher parties. At the time of departure of those first three casualties, he had probably decided who were the next three casualties on the priority list and the next three after them, etc. However, this should not be an inflexible decision, because by the time the stretcher parties return, the situation could have changed, since one person's general condition may have deteriorated more rapidly than expected in relation to the general conditions of the other casualties. This can happen because we are all individuals and not machines. Some people have a physical resilience which others do not, and so as individuals, we respond to injury each in our own individual way. For this reason the Chief First Aider cannot afford to relax until all the casualties have been evacuated. He should instruct his First Aiders to monitor the general condition of the non-walking casualties until they are evacuated by checking regularly on facial appearance, pulse, pupils (in head injuries), respiration, temperature and (if possible) blood pressure, preferably every fifteen minutes. By this stage of the operation, the non-walking casualties should include any of the walking casualties who have been singled out because of suspected internal injuries. Having deployed his First Aiders to the task of monitoring the remaining non-walking casualties, the Chief First Aider can check around to see if his order of priority of evacuation is still correct or whether it needs to be changed.

I will end this chapter and this book by reminding you that a person with multiple injuries will die unless he receives a blood transfusion. However, I pointed out in Part I that ECF (extracellular fluid) is the human equivalent of the hump on the camel's back, and that ECF can be used to replace the *volume* of blood lost, and thus it buys time for the injured person. Also I pointed out that this time is valuable, because ECF is not blood and there is a limit to the time a person can stay alive with a grossly depleted supply of red blood cells.

So my advice to every First Aider is that you should not waste time, because *time means life*. Therefore you should practise examination on each other as described in Part II, so that when the time comes, you can secure the airway, stop bleeding (except that from inside the ear) diagnose the injuries quickly, splint and bandage *adequately* and then get on with evacuation as soon as possible. As long as your splinting and bandaging are *functional* it does not matter if they do not look beautiful. So do not spend too much time splinting and bandaging because a beautifully splinted corpse is not an achievement of which you can be proud! The sooner the injured person arrives at hospital, where blood is available, the sooner his chances of survival will improve.

Glossary

Air hunger. This is deep, sighing respiration. It is caused by gross loss of red blood cells.

Amnesia. This is loss of memory (i.e. inability to recall facts or events).

   a. *Anterograde amnesia* is loss of memory for events after a head injury (i.e. going forward in time from the time of the injury). It includes any period of unconsciousness.

   b. *Retrograde amnesia* is loss of memory for events prior to a head injury. The duration of retrograde amnesia is *directly* proportional to the severity of the head injury.

Apnoea. This means that a person is not breathing.

Apoplexy. This is commonly called a 'Stroke'. It is sometimes referred to as a cerebrovascular accident, or CVA for brevity. Examples are cerebral haemorrhage, cerebral thrombosis and subarachnoid haemorrhage.

Asphyxia. This is a condition in which the blood is grossly under-oxygenated. Its causes may be either physical or chemical. If the cause is not eliminated quickly enough, the victim of asphyxia will die.

Automatism. This is a condition, which may occur after an epileptic fit, and which may last up to twenty-four hours. It is characterised by the performance of routine, or automatic, actions, e.g. going for a bus ride on a certain bus route, or going to a certain cinema, or going for a walk on a specific route. In other words, these automatic actions have a definite pattern.

Braxton-Hicks contractions. These are *painless* contractions of the womb, which occur during the last twelve weeks of pregnancy. They indicate that the womb is toning itself up for labour.

Cheyne-Stokes respiration. This is a form of respiration characterised by 'crescendos' of breathing interspersed with periods of apnoea (no breathing). It should *not* be confused with high-altitude respiration.

Compression of the brain. This is a condition caused by continuous bleeding inside the skull. The bleeding forms an ever-enlarging pool of blood within the skull. In turn, this ever-enlarging pool of blood exerts a continuous and ever-increasing pressure on the brain, inside the skull. Thus, the brain is gradually *compressed* by the enlarging pool of blood, within an inexpandible bony box (the skull). This condition should *not* be confused with a *depressed* skull fracture.

Concussion. This simply means brain damage. It is diagnosed from the history of a head injury, which has resulted in *retrograde* amnesia.

CSF. This is an abbreviation for cerebrospinal fluid. It is a crystal-clear fluid, which bathes the central nervous system (the brain and spinal cord). It lies between the brain and spinal cord, on the one hand, and their coverings (the meninges) on the other.

Diastole. This is the period, during which the heart relaxes.

Dislocation. This is defined as 'complete loss of apposition of the surfaces of a joint'.

ECF. This is extracellular fluid. Strictly speaking, it includes blood, CSF, the interstitial fluid and lymph – i.e. all the body fluids, which are *outside* the cells of the body. *For the purposes of the text of this book only*, ECF refers to the interstitial fluid – i.e. the fluid which lies between the bloodstream and the cells.

Effusion. This is an excessive amount of synovial fluid, or blood, or both, within a synovial joint. Usually, an effusion occurs as a result of injury. Sometimes, an effusion may be caused by disease or infection. In the case of infection, the effusion is quite likely to contain pus.

Embolism. This is the blocking of a blood vessel by a sufficiently large particle (or *embolus*) carried along by the bloodstream. Embolism commonly causes *infarction* (i.e. death) of the tissues supplied by the blocked blood-vessel, e.g. myocardial infarction is the death of part of the heart muscle (or myocardium).

Embolus. This is the particle which causes an embolism. It may be (a) a detached blood clot, (b) detached, infected 'vegetations', from a diseased heart valve, (c) a fat embolus, which can occur after multiple fractures, or after the fracture of a large bone, or (d) an air embolus, which may occur accidentally, during an intravenous infusion of fluid, or during a blood transfusion. The commonest form of embolus is a detached blood clot.

Excretion. This is the process, by which unwanted by-products of metabolism are removed from the body.

Haematoma. This is a collection of blood in an unusual position within the body, but outside the bloodstream. It usually occurs as a result of injury, but can occur spontaneously in certain diseases (e.g. Leukaemia).

Haemothorax. This is a collection of blood within the chest, or thorax. In effect, it is a haematoma inside the chest. The collection of blood lies between the lung and the chest wall. It is usually the result of an injury to the chest.

ICF. This is intracellular fluid – i.e. the fluid inside the body cells.

Infarct. *see* **Embolism.**

Liquor. (pronounced, 'Lie-kwor'). This is a crystal-clear, rather sweet-smelling liquid. It bathes and protects an unborn baby inside the sac of membranes within the womb. This liquor should not be confused with alcoholic liquor (pronounced, 'Likkor').

Meninges. These are the coverings of the central nervous system (the brain and spinal cord).

Meniscus. (plural = menisci). This is a new-moon-shaped structure. There are two in each knee joint and their function is to facilitate rotational movements in the flexed, or semi-flexed, knee joint. They are commonly referred to as 'cartilages'. The TM joints also have menisci, to facilitate lateral (sideways) movements of the lower jaw.

Metabolic rate. This is the *rate* at which energy is produced and used.

Metabolism. This word means the production and use of energy.

Midclavicular line. This is an imaginary line, drawn perpendicularly from the midpoint of the clavicle, on either side. Since this line usually passes through the nipple, it is often called the 'nipple line'.

Movements. These are fetal movements, i.e. the movements of an unborn baby inside the womb. The mother may start to feel them any time from the sixteenth week of pregnancy onwards.

Muscle-spasm. This occurs after injury, reflexly. It reduces movement at the site of injury, which, in turn, reduces pain. It is Nature's own built-in, self-splinting mechanism.

Myocardial infarct. This is the death of all, or part, of the heart muscle. (*see* **Embolism**).

Neck rigidity. This means that the neck cannot be flexed so that the chin touches the chest. It occurs typically in meningitis, encephalitis and subarachnoid haemorrhage.

Oedema. This is a localised, excessive collection of tissue fluid. The fluid is interspersed amongst the cells locally. Typically, a 'pitting', or 'pitmark', can be made in oedema by pressing with a finger for about five seconds. This 'pitting' distinguishes oedema from a haematoma, which does not 'pit'. Oedema commonly results from injury. It may occur in association with fractures, where the bone lies just under the skin (e.g. skull, clavicle, ulna and tibia). When oedema of the scalp occurs, after a head injury, it is virtually always diagnostic of a fracture of the skull and it marks the fracture site. Oedema may also occur (a) in the feet, ankles and legs of a person, who is suffering from congestive heart failure and (b) locally, at the site of an acute infection (e.g. a boil or an abscess).

Olecranon process. This is the upper end of the ulna. Together with the upper end of the radius and the lower end of the humerus, it forms the elbow joint.

Opiates. These are drugs derived from Opium, which comes from the opium poppy. Typical examples are Pethidine, Morphine, Papaveretum ('Omnopon') and Diamorphine ('Heroin').

Peritoneum. This is the inner lining of the abdomen. It is rather sensitive to irritation, pain, etc.

Reactive hyperaemia. This is an excessive dilatation of the blood vessels of the skin. It occurs after a period of constriction of the blood vessels (e.g. in response to a very cold environment).

Retroperitoneal haematoma. (*see* 'Haematoma'). This is a haematoma, which lies behind the peritoneum (the inner lining of the abdomen), but in front of the muscles, which cover the front of the lumbar spine. It results from injury, and can account for between two and four pints of blood loss.

Rigidity. This is the term used to describe muscle-spasm in the abdomen. It may occur in response to injury, or to disease (e.g. acute appendicitis, or perforated duodenal ulcer).

Shock. This is a clinical condition, characterised by pallor, a cold, clammy skin and a rapid, thready pulse. These three signs are always associated with a lowered blood pressure. (for types of shock, *see* text, p. 22).

Show. This is a blood-stained, mucus plug, which is released from the neck of the womb, either prior to labour, or during the first stage of labour.

Sign. This is something, which is found on examination of a person.

Situs inversus. This is a condition in which the apex beat of the heart is to be found in the right side of the chest, instead of in the left side of the chest, as in normal people. People, who have situs inversus, are usually quite healthy. In *complete situs inversus*, each organ is to be found in the opposite side of the body to that in which it is normally found (e.g. spleen on the right, appendix on the left). In fact, the whole of the body is a 'mirror image' of the normal arrangement of the human body.

Status epilepticus. This is a series of epileptic fits strung together – i.e. before one fit is completed, another fit begins, etc. If not treated promptly, it can be fatal.

Stroke. *see* **Apoplexy.**

Subluxation. This is defined as 'incomplete loss of apposition of the surfaces of a joint'.

Surgical emphysema. This is air in the soft tissues of the front of the neck. On palpation, it gives a soft, crinkly, tissue-paper-like feeling to the fingers. It results from a severe compression injury to the chest.

Symptom. This is something of which a patient complains, e.g. pain, inability to walk, etc.

Synovial fluid. This is the fluid produced by the synovial membrane (the delicate inner lining) of a synovial joint. It lubricates the joint surfaces.

Systole. This is the period, during which the heart is contracting – i.e. pumping out blood.

Thrombosis. This is the formation of a blood clot, or thrombus. It usually occurs in a vein, but can occur in one of the coronary arteries, which supply the heart muscle, in which case a coronary thrombosis, or myocardial infarct, occurs. (*see* **Infarct**).

Uraemia. This is a condition, in which there is a gross build-up of urea and ammonia in the blood. It is indicative of serious kidney disease.

Urea. This is a harmless by-product of protein breakdown. Urea is excreted by the kidneys.

Uterus. This organ is commonly referred to as the womb. It serves as an incubator and as protection for an unborn baby during pregnancy, and its muscle provides the expulsive force required during labour.

Zygomatic arch. This is the bony arch, which can be felt, as it passes from the cheek-bone to just in front of the ear. There is one arch on each side of the face. These arches help to preserve the normal facial contours.

Index